Research Appreciation:
*An Initial Guide for Nurses
and Health Care
Professionals*

Central Health Studies:

The Central Health Studies (CHS) series is designed to provide nurses and other health care professionals with up-to-date, informative texts on key professional and management issues and human skills in health care.

The Consulting Editor:

The series was conceived by John Tingle, BA Law Hons, Cert Ed, M Ed, Barrister, Senior Lecturer in Law, Nottingham Law School, Nottingham Polytechnic. John has published widely on the subject of the professional and legal accountability of health care professionals.

Other Books in the Series

Spiritual Care: A Resource Guide

Budgeting Skills: A Guide for Nurse Managers

Portfolio Development and Profiling for Nurses

Patients' Rights, Responsibilities and the Nurse

Measuring the Effectiveness of Nurse Education: The use of performance indicators

Employment Law for Nurses

Central Health Studies
Consulting Editor: John Tingle

Research Appreciation:

An Initial Guide for Nurses and Health Care Professionals

**Paula McGee
and Joy Notter**

Quay Books Division of Mark Allen Publishing Limited
Jesses Farm, Snow Hill, Dinton, Nr Salisbury, Wilts, SP3 5HN

©Mark Allen Publishing Ltd, 1995

British Library Cataloguing-in-Publication Data
A catalogue record for this book is available from the British Library

ISBN 1-85642-026-4

All rights reserved. No part of this material may be reproduced, stored in a retrieval system, or transmitted in any form, or by any means, electrical, mechanical, photographic, recording, or otherwise, without the prior permission of the publishers.

Printed and bound in Great Britain by
Biddles Ltd, Guildford and King's Lynn

CONTENTS

Introduction: Is research for you? vii

Chapter One:
What is research? 1

Chapter Two:
What do you want to know? 11

Chapter Three:
How do you find out? 27

Chapter Four:
Whom can you ask? 43

Chapter Five:
Will people agree to take part? 55

Chapter Six:
What can you find out? 63

Chapter Seven:
What can you do with your data? 83

Chapter Eight:
How do you interpret interviews and
observations? 119

Chapter Nine:
How do you write about your findings? 131

Chapter Ten:
Glossary of research terms 137

Appendix: Referencing your work 143

Abbreviations 147

Index 149

Introduction:

Is research for you?

Nursing in the real world, as opposed to the ideal presented in many nursing texts, is a mixture of many things - hard physical work, conflicting demands, tradition,"Sister likes it this way", local policies, rapid decision making, constant change and little time to think! In the midst of all this it must sometimes seem a miracle that any of our patients recover from their illnesses or progress towards peaceful deaths (Henderson 1960), yet many do so. The question is – *how*? Most of the time we are so busy just keeping our heads above water that we are scarcely aware of what we do, let alone how we do it. Yet that awareness is crucial in the provision of any health service today. The essence of the separation of purchasers from providers in health service management is that for the first time those, such as nurses, who provide services must specify the nature of their services to potential customers, or purchasers, and devise a realistic set of charges. If nurses cannot do this for themselves, the current wisdom is that someone else will do it for them and sell them short. In other words, **"If at the end of the day you cannot tell others what you have been doing, then your doing has been in vain"** (Schrodinger 1951).

Tackling this situation means asking searching questions about both what patients want and the nature of nursing activity. The answers may be painful. We may have to give up some cherished practices that we have carefully nurtured over the years but on the other hand there is hope that some of what we do may be vindicated and that new practices will emerge based on a sound knowledge base in nursing rather than tradition alone.

Asking questions, finding answers, introducing change - this is the stuff of research. Research is about finding out; about finding ways to make things happen. Nursing has traditionally suffered from the view that research is something separate from other nursing work. For example, during pre-Registration training most of us were taught by people who did not acknowledge any research basis for their teaching. Research was a separate topic on the

Research appreciation

timetable, an ivory tower of little relevance to the real business of nursing and consequently it seemed our tutors knew everything as if by magic. Modern nursing curricula are attempting to address this situation and the National Boards for Nursing are quite explicit in their expectations of nurses entering the Register. The Boards expect nurses to be able to critically evaluate research reports and to utilise research findings appropriately in practice.

This book is intended to help you achieve these expectations and, if you wish, to move beyond them and undertake a research project. It is essentially a self help package with a number of excercises designed to introduce you to each stage of the research process. These excercises can be used by you alone, by small groups of approximately six people or alongside formal teaching or research. We aim to demystify research and research activities thus making them accessible to a wide range of practitioners. The book:

- **outlines** the whole of the research process
- **identifies** the skills needed to undertake research and who might be able to help you
- **helps** you express research questions clearly
- **explains** research terms both in the text and in the glossary
- **explains** the steps involved in planning a research project
- **explains** the steps involved in undertaking a research project
- **helps** you develop strategies you can use to introduce research findings into practice.
- **outlines** the ways in which you can use your research project in terms of academic or career development.

The book is intended as an introduction to research primarily for those nurses working in the field of nursing **practice**. Ideas for further development or reading are given at the end of each chapter.

References

Henderson V (1960). *Basic Priciples of Nursing Care* International Council of Nurses, Geneva

Schrodinger E (1951). Science and Humanism Cambridge University Press, Cambridge, in Zukav G (1991) *The Dancing Wu Li Masters Rider*, 2 edn, Rider, London

Chapter 1
What is Research?

Introduction

At the end of this chapter you will be able to:

i) identify and briefly explain the stages of the research process
ii) briefly explain some of the terminology used in the research process.
iii) begin to plan a research project

Research is essentially about finding out; discovering new ideas; trying out different approaches to a problem. The key element within these activities is science. Research is a scientific process and it is this which distinguishes it from other lines of enquiry.

Getting started

This chapter will give you an overview of the entire research process so that you have a picture of how it all hangs together. It will introduce some new terminology which will be explained briefly at this point and in more detail in the glossary of terms. Each stage of the research process will be explained in more detail in subsequent chapters.

The research process

The research process has several distinct stages.

1. The research question

According to Bronowski (1973) this *"is the essence of science: ask an impertinent question and you are on the way to a pertinent answer."* The research question is the focus of the entire research project. Whatever the subject being investigated the research question must be as clear as possible. Achieving this is not as easy as it sounds and some guidelines on how to develop clear research questions are set out in chapter two.

The research question can be expressed in different ways:

***An hypothesis*:** This is a statement which requires to be proved or disproved.

Examples might include:

> *There is a positive relationship between nurses' perceptions of their workload and their decisions to change jobs.*
>
> *Turning unconscious patients every two hours prevents pressure sore formation.*

A research question: This is a direct question which may emerge as the hypothesis develops or, as in this instance, it may stand alone. It enables the researcher to discover relationships without the additional elements of proof or disproof which may sometimes be impossible to achieve. A research question might be appropriate for a small scale study.

Examples might include:

> *What do nurses understand about the action of Granuflex?*
>
> *How do nurses plan the discharge of a patient who has had a stroke?*

A research statement: This indicates that the research is descriptive or evaluative in nature rather than seeking to answer questions or prove an hypothesis.

Examples might include:

> *An evaluation of the preparation of student nurses for transcultural care settings.*
>
> *The development of new practices in Health Visiting.*

2. The literature review

This is a thorough review of the literature relevant to the subject being researched. It is based on a systematic search using library sources and involves the researcher recording and summarising what s/he has read; critically reviewing what has been read and identifying themes. The object is to enable the researcher to both develop insight into the subject area as a basis for the project and to place the project within the context of research to date.

3. Method

This stage involves a number of steps. First, the aims and objectives of the research must be clearly identified.

The type of **data** (information) which might help achieve these aims and objectives will be examined. Data may be classified in different ways but in simple terms it may be seen as **objective and quantitative** (concerned with measurement, establishing the relationships between selected factors) or **subjective and qualitative** (concerned with seeking to understand peoples' experiences of the world), (Cohen and Manion 1989). Each type of data has its' strengths and weaknesses and the ultimate selection of quantitative or qualitative data as a basis for the research depends on a number of factors based on different ways of looking at the world and the particular topic to be researched.

First of all the researcher has to consider *'Is this topic something which occurs in people's minds? Is it about the way they think or feel or do I think this topic is outside the person and, therefore, outside what happens in their mind?'* Consideration of these

ontological perspectives (Burrell and Morgan 1979) will help the researcher recognise that some topics may be better researched by specifically gathering quantitative data or qualitative data, or a mixture of both (triangulation, Denzin 1989).

Secondly, the researcher must consider the nature of knowledge and the forms it takes (**epistemological perspectives**). Here, the researcher might ask '*Is knowledge something hard, tangible based on facts or is it something more fluid based perhaps, on experience or insight?*' In addition to the researcher's own answers, it is necessary to acknowledge that each profession defines knowledge in its' own way (Chinn and Kramer 1991). For example medical knowledge is defined very much in terms of the physical and biological sciences; as hard, factual information. Nursing knowledge, on the other hand, is less easy to define as it is based on both science and human interaction. Thirdly, the researcher must consider the **interrelationship between people and their environment**. Human behaviour will always be influenced by environmental factors, be they natural or artificial, which may vary from day to day (Burrell and Morgan 1979).

Having selected the type of data most appropriate for the study the researcher must consider the method or methods which might be suitable for the study. Examples of these methods are interviews, questionnaires, observation. Each method has advantages and disadvantages and the researcher must select the one or ones most likely to yield results. If no one method is likely to be completely suitable, it may be appropriate to use a technique called triangulation in which a combination of methods is employed (Denzin, 1989).

The sources of the data are considered with regard to their suitability for the research. Sources might include patients, staff, colleagues, records, relatives etc. Having decided which sources to use the researcher then constructs a smaller group or **sample**. Chapter 4 will show you how this is done.

Alongside these matters the researcher must recognise the ethical dimensions of what s/he is planning to do. The study of ethics is the critical evaluation of assumptions and arguments about 'norms', 'values', 'right and wrong', 'good and bad' and 'what ought and ought not to be done' (Gillon 1985). In this context the researcher must ask *"Is it acceptable to do this (method) to people?"* These issues are discussed further in Chapter 4.

4. Data collection

The data is collected. The different methods of data collection are set out in Chapter 6.

5. Data analysis

The data is analysed with reference to the aims and objectives of the study. Guidelines on how to do this are set out in Chapters 7 and 8.

6. Discussion of the findings and forming conclusions

This stage draws the various elements of the research together. The results of the analysis are discussed critically with reference to the literature review. The researcher must determine whether the analysis of the data supports or contradicts the work of others and the possible reasons for this. Similarly the methods used must be critically evaluated in the light of the research. The researcher must consider whether, with hindsight, the methods used were the most suitable and if they proved to be flawed, the possible reasons for this. From this discussion conclusions will emerge together with recommendations for further study if appropriate.

7. Sharing the findings of the research

The final stage must be to share the the findings with others - to publish in a journal or circulate a report to as many colleagues as possible. Research which is simply left to gather dust is worthless but often nurses are concerned that their study is somehow '*not good enough*' to publish. Something may not have gone according to plan, the results were not conclusive or the study was very small. Whatever the perceived defects it is still worth sharing. There is probably no such thing as the perfect research project. If perfect research was possible, human knowledge would probably advance far more quickly and research, itself, would be easy. The reality is that in every study there will be some flaw, something imperfect and maybe by sharing your findings rather than keeping them to yourself, someone else may have ideas which will help you.

Looking at the research process overall, it may seem a daunting task but the scale or size of a project can vary greatly depending on what the researcher is aiming to achieve. The project can be as large or as small as you wish and the remainder of this chapter gives some guidelines for planning a project. This plan is called a **protocol**. It should be brief - about 1500-2000 words at the most.

Guidelines for a research protocol

The protocol should have the following sections:

a) the research question and the aims and objectives of the project (see Chapter 2.)

b) a brief statement of the issues associated with the the subject you wish to research and how you have come to be concerned about it. (see Chapter 2)

c) a brief overview of the method you plan to use. (See Chapter 4).

d) identification of the ethical issues involved (See Chapter 5).

e) a statement of resources required and the costs involved (see Chapter 2).

f) a table showing the time scale of the project. (See Chapter 2).

g) a brief statement about how the project will be monitored.

An example of a research protocol

Research Statement

An evaluation of the service provided by District Nurses to elderly clients.

Aim: The overall aims of this study are to provide an evaluation of the service provided to elderly clients by District Nurses.

Objectives: To achieve this aim the researcher will:
- i) undertake a comprehensive review of the relevant literature.
- ii) critically evaluate the views of clients with regard to the quality and effectiveness of the service.
- iii) critically evaluate the views of carers with regard to the quality and effectiveness of the service.
- iv) synthesise the above findings.
- v) produce a report outlining the findings of the research, the conclusions drawn and the recommendations for the future.

Issues in this project

There is a growing number of elderly clients. Many of these clients have multiple problems and rely on a network of support services, including social services, district nurses etc., to meet their needs. Inevitably, some overlap occurs between the services and there is a need to clarify some of the activities which contribute to this overlap.

As yet no systematic enquiry has been undertaken into the degree of client and carer satisfaction with regard to the District Nurse Service.

In addition, it is not entirely clear what duties should be the preserve of the District Nurse and what can safely be left to others.

Choice of research methods

The numbers of clients and carers is large and the research aims to reach as many people as possible in order to elicit their views. The methods chosen must, therefore, be suitable for use with large numbers and a survey approach seems most appropriate. it has also to be remembered that some people may prefer to be anonymous whilst others may not be able to complete a questionnaire because of some form of disability. The method must both protect the identity of individuals and allow others to make their views heard.

The tools used in the survey will be:
- questionnaire to all clients
- questionnaire to all carers

The researcher will arrange to visit those clients who cannot complete the questionnaire, read each question to them and note their answers.

The sample

As the aim of this project is to provide a comprehensive evaluation of the work of the district nurse the sample for the study will be all the elderly people and their carers who are currently receiving a service from the district nurses in this health authority. Although this will mean a large sample, it will provide an opportunity for all recipients of the service, including those with communication difficulties, to air their views.

Ethical Issues

Access to subjects

Permission to approach clients and their carers to ask them to take part in the study will be negotiated via the Health Authority's Ethics Committee and the appropriate managers.

Recruitment and Consent

Each potential participant will be given written and verbal information about the project and asked if they would agree to participate. Those who do agree will be asked to sign a consent form. They will be assured that their identity and any data they give will be confidential and used only for the purposes of the project.

Resources

The researcher will require:	Estimated cost
Time	
Word processing facilities	
Library Facilities	
Postage costs	
Telephone costs	
Travel costs	
The total cost is estimated as.....	

Time scale

The project will take place over a period of eight months

	Completed by
Approval from ethics committee and managers	month 1
Literature search	month 2
Questionnaires designed and tested	month 3
Questionnaires sent out	month 4
Questionnaires returned and analysed	month 5 & 6
Report written	month 7 & 8

Management of the Project

The progress of the project will be monitored and reviewed at intervals throughout its' duration. This will be achieved by meetings between the researcher, and a more experienced researcher who acts as **supervisor.** The supervisor's role will be to act as a sounding board for ideas, advise on appropriate action and generally guide the researcher. This is not to say that the researcher is in any way undermined. It is the researcher who is responsible for the project and who, at the end of the day, must decide whether to accept the advice and guidance offered by the supervisor.

Conclusion

This chapter has introduced you to the research process and shown you how to plan a project. The remainder of this book is intended to help you develop your knowledge and skill with regard to research.

References

Bronowski J (1973). *The Ascent of Man*, Science Horizons Inc. and BBC Publications, London.

Burrell G and Morgan G (1979). *Sociological Paradigms and Organisational Analysis,* Heinemann, London

Chinn P and Kramer M (1991). *Theory and Nursing 3rd edn.* Mosby Year Book, St. Louis.

Cohen L and Manion L (1989). *Research Methods in Education 3rd edn.* Routledge, London

Denzin N (1989). *The Research Act 3rd edn.* Prentice Hall, Englewood Cliffs, New Jersey

Gillon R (1985). *Philosophical Medical Ethics,* John Wiley and Sons, Chichester.

Chapter 2
What Do You Want to Know?

Introduction

At the end of this chapter you will be able to:

i) develop a clear research question for a project

ii) clearly state some of the issues associated with that research question

iii) quantify the resources you require for your project including funding.

In addition this chapter will provide some information about developing your knowledge of research through courses in higher education.

Identifying clearly what it is you want to know is the most crucial and difficult part of the research process. It is crucial because it underpins all subsequent activities. If you have not thought out clearly what you want to know you are more likely to get side-tracked, become overwhelmed by too much information or quite simply to get stuck. The chance of you then completing the project and discovering the answers to the questions which concern you are then greatly reduced. However, expressing clearly what you want to know is not always easy. Problems rarely exist in isolation but in a state of inter-relatedness to each other. Moreover, problems are often complex and multifaceted. Easy solutions may not be apparent – hence the need for research.

This chapter is presented as a series of steps, each of which is timed to help you structure the activities involved. The steps should be followed in sequence. Don't worry if you take less than the recommended time or if you take a little longer but if steps 1 - 3 last for more than 1 1/2 hours you may be trying to cram too much in at this stage. If this situation develops take **one** aspect of the

Research appreciation

problem only and repeat step 1 concentrating only on that. Narrowing down the focus of attention may help to separate the proverbial wood from the trees!

STEP 1   **"BRAINSTORMING"**

TIME REQUIRED: APPROXIMATELY 20 MINUTES

Let's start by making yourself comfortable away from the direct working environment and minimising interruptions (including the telephone). A not too busy late shift would be ideal for this . You will need a pen and paper as well as peace and quiet. During the next twenty minutes give the "problem" your full attention. Begin by expressing it in your own words in the middle of the page (Fig.1) From this central point draw lines radiating outwards (Fig.1) and beside each jot down anything that comes into your mind about the "problem". Questions which might help to get you started on this include:

> *What do I think is causing this problem?*
>
> *When does it occur?*
>
> *Who is involved?*
>
> *What are the effects of this problem?*
>
> *What solutions have been tried so far?*
>
> *What were the results?*

Try not to think too hard at this stage. This may seem a strange piece of advice but just letting ideas flow, or "brainstorming" even apparently daft suggestions, can sometimes help to unlock aspects of the problem that have not been considered before. In a group, "brainstorming" also provides an opportunity for people to let off

What do you want to know?

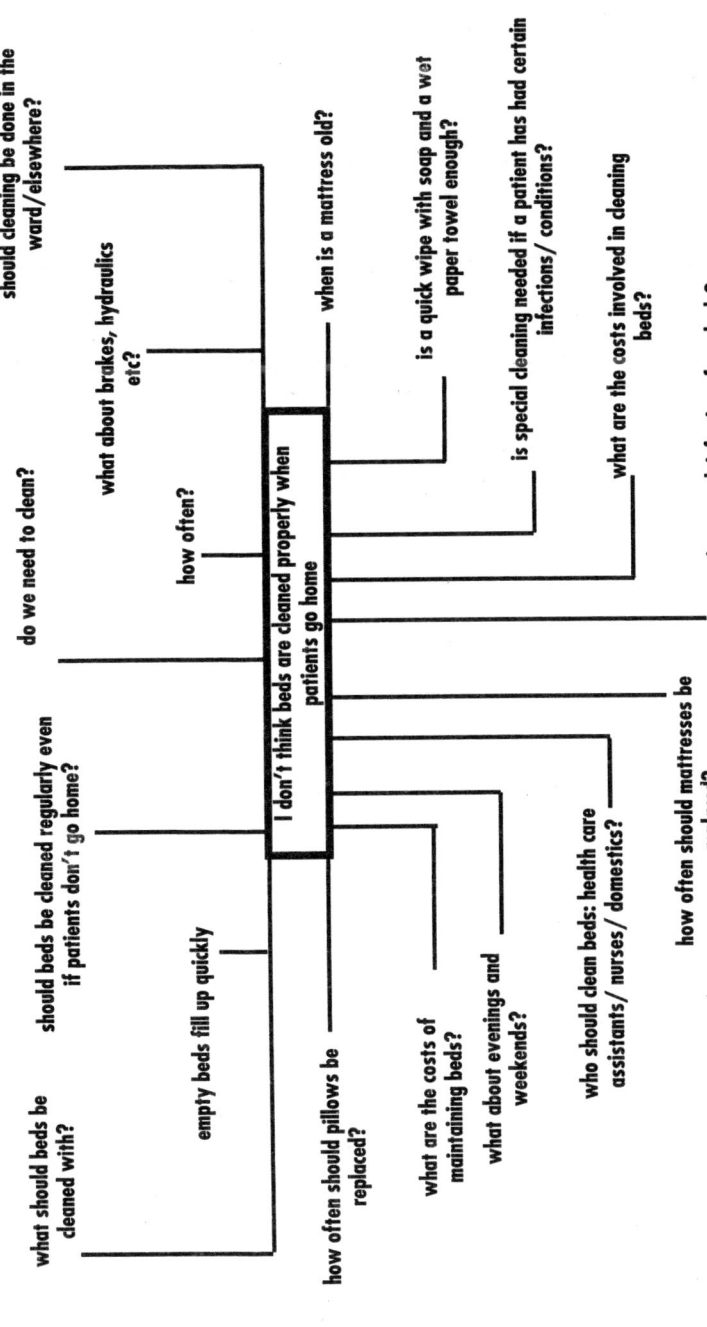

Figure 2.1: Brainstorming

Research appreciation

STEP 2

PRIORITISING

TIME REQUIRED: APPROXIMATELY 15 MINUTES

steam about a particular problem which can have the effect of releasing frustrations and clearing the mind as well as the air.

Look at the brainstorming you have done so far and, using a different coloured pen, place a [1] beside those points you consider to be most relevant to the problem (Fig. 2). Then, using a different colour, place a [2] beside those you consider to be less relevant but still related to the problem. In the next category identify those points which have very little relevance with a [3]. As you approach each point explain briefly why you are putting it in a particular group.

By grouping points together it is possible to see issues emerging which require further investigation and others which you may wish to lay aside.

Points coded as 1:

- Do we need to clean?
- What should beds be cleaned with?
- Is a quick wipe with soap and a wet paper towel enough?
- Is special cleaning needed if a patient has has certain infections/conditions?
- What are the costs involved in cleaning beds?
- Empty beds fill up so quickly.
- Should beds be cleaned regularly even if the patient does not go home?

What do you want to know?

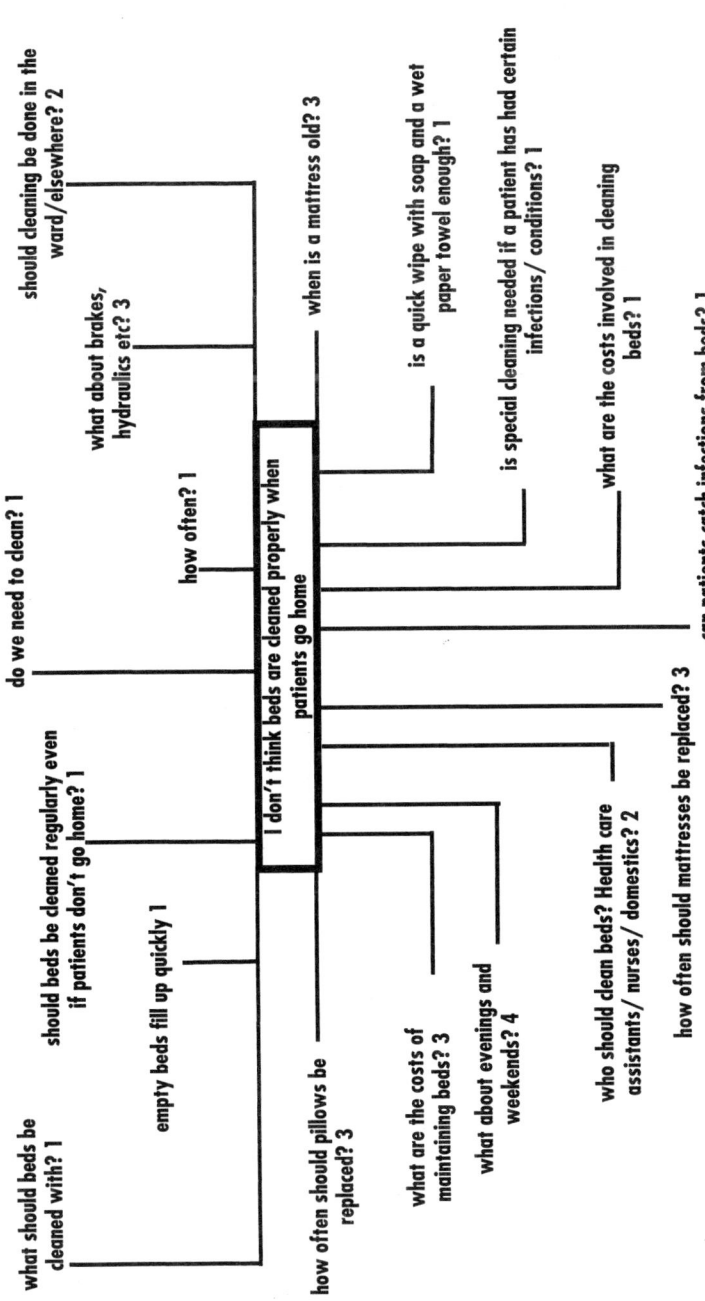

Figure 2.2: Prioritising

Research appreciation

- How often?
- Can patients catch infections from beds?

All of these questions relate directly to some aspect of bed cleaning and, in the real world, would be supplemented by individuals' comments and opinions which would have emerged during the brainstorming session.

Points coded as 2:

- Should cleaning be done in the ward or elsewhere?
- Who should clean beds - Health Care Assistants/Nurses/Domestics?

It might be possible to include these amongst the items in the previous group but these two points do not relate specifically to the actual cleaning of beds but rather to where they should be cleaned and by whom. It would be possible to spend a lot of time discussing these matters and lose sight of the original problem. In such a situation **you** have to decide whether you wish to include them in the number 1 priority group, deal with them as separate issues perhaps in another project, or abandon them altogether.

Points coded as 3:

- What about the brakes, hydraulics etc?
- How often should pillows be replaced?
- What are the costs of maintaining beds?
- When is a mattress old?

Each of these points moves further away from the subject of cleaning beds and it would be best to leave them aside for another project.

Points coded as 4:

- What about evenings and weekends?

Well what about them? The question does not seem to have much relevance to anything discussed so far and, as it is not even very clear what is intended, can be abandoned.

What do you want to know?

One final point:

> **don't throw away your notes!**

No matter how untidy or messy you think they look, keep them. Firstly, they will be a reminder of your original ideas. As your research progresses you will come across many new and novel ideas; collect a lot of information from many different sources; sometimes wonder if it is all worth it and if you are going in the right direction. In short, when you are up to your neck in alligators you will need something to remind you that your first intention was to drain the swamp!

Just as important is the need to be able to show others how you have arrived at your conclusions at the end of your project. Other people must be able to see where you started out from; how your ideas developed; why you did certain things and not others; all the steps involved in your discoveries. Ideally, another researcher should be able to replicate your research and achieve similar results.

STEP 3

MAKING A STATEMENT

TIME REQUIRED: APPROXIMATELY 10-15 MINUTES

Look again at the points coded 1.

> *I don't think that beds are cleaned properly when patients go home.*
> - Do we need to clean?
> - What should beds be cleaned with?
> - Is a quick wipe with soap and a wet paper towel enough?
> - Is special cleaning needed if a patient has has certain infections/conditions?

Research appreciation

- What are the costs involved in cleaning beds?
- Empty beds fill up so quickly.
- Should beds be cleaned regularly even if the patient does not go home?
- How often?
- Can patients catch infections from beds?

At this stage you need to review this list and, drawing on the ideas included in it, try to re-express what you want to know in a single sentence to form a research question (Chapter 1) and identify from your brainstorming the relevant points or issues. Examples might include:

Hypothesis

- Washing with soap and water when the patient is discharged is enough to clean any bed.

Issues

- Nurses are currently using an array of different substances to clean beds. These cost money and are probably unnecessary. Saving money on bed cleaning may help provide funds for something else.

Research Question

- Is there a relationship between the cleanliness of beds and infections in patients?

Issues

- Many of the beds and mattresses used are quite old. Other items in the ward environment are known sources of infection. Little attention has so far been paid to whether beds can carry infection.

Research Statement

- A comparison of the effects of cleaning beds with two different cleaning agents.

Issues

- Nurses are currently using an array of different substances to clean beds but little is known about the effectiveness of them. Saving money on bed cleaning may help provide funds for something else.

STEP 4

CHECKING OUT YOUR IDEAS

TIME REQUIRED: VARIABLE BUT ALLOW AT LEAST 2/3 DAYS

When you have completed this exercise leave the matter alone for a few days. During that time try to find opportunities to talk to others about your ideas. Talking through your ideas, explaining what you want to find out particularly to people who have not been involved so far will help to clarify your research question further.

Developing a clear research question is not the only issue. A major concern at this stage must be *'is the question worth asking?'* Last year a friend of the author described her experiences of participating in a research project. A researcher came to her house and interviewed her at great length. *"What exactly are you trying to find out?"* asked the woman. *"Why married women get depressed?"* came the reply. The woman laughed and said, *"But I could have told you that in five minutes! I have five young children. We have to constantly struggle to make ends meet. My husband works long hours. Of course I get depressed!"* It may be that the researcher did not explain things very well but the main point here is that to the participant, the research seemed a waste of time as the answer was, to her, quite obvious. There are two ways of looking at this story.

The "so what?" factor

Is the answer to your research question really worth knowing? In the final analysis of course only you can answer that but, in doing so, you may have to be brutally honest and acknowledge that what you thought was a good idea is really a waste of time. Research must have some practical purpose in extending the basis of nursing knowledge. As Medawar (1967) points out there is sometimes a case for a *"free ranging inquiry"* which has no immediate application but which will lead, it is hoped, to *"something practically useful"*. However, he goes on to suggest that:

> *"Might not the converse approach be equally effective .... to start with a concrete problem but then to allow the research to open out in the direction of greater generality, so that the more particular and special discoveries can be made to rank as theorems."*

The **'ivory tower'** approach to research is, therefore, not necessary. It should be possible to begin with a practical issue of direct relevance to patient care.

Is the obvious really so clear?

It has to be acknowledged that this is frequently not the case. To believe otherwise is to tread the path of fatalism - that things will happen anyway. Fatalism results in the perpetuation of outmoded practice because the 'obvious' reason for acting in a particular way is never challenged. Walsh and Ford (1989), amongst others, have tried to draw nurses' attention to this situation. They cite, for example, the subject of pre-operative care in which it is 'obvious' that patients must be shaved yet it has been demonstrated that depilatory creams are associated positively with a lower post operative infection rate than that which occurs following shaving (Lancet editorial 1983; Winfield 1986). Moreover depilation is quicker, cheaper and less embarrassing for the patient. In another example, it is 'obvious' that patients' rings should be removed prior to surgery but

> *"why do we remove all a patient's rings except the wedding ring? Are wedding rings in some way repellent to bacteria but other plain metal rings are not? Given that the ring may have remained on the person's finger for fifty years and never been taken off, why do we tape it on then go to theatre as if afraid that it will jump off at the sight of a scalpel?"*
>
> (Walsh and Ford 1989).

STEP 5

IDENTIFYING RESOURCES FOR THE PROJECT

Now that you have a clear idea for a project in mind, it is worth spending some time identifying the resources you may need to undertake it **before** you get too involved. There are a number of important points to consider at this stage:

i) "I feel strongly about this issue"

Good! Research that doesn't interest you can only be described as a chore. There has to be some sense of interest and a feeling of commitment to the project in order to see it through especially when things get difficult. Feelings, however, are not enough to produce good quality work nor should they be allowed to cloud your judgement. Good quality research seeks to be objective in amassing data and constructing arguments which are based on intellectual rather than emotional foundations. Very strong preconceived ideas could lead to your concentrating more on evidence which supports your views and less on that which contradicts them.

ii) "Care must be research based"

Yes it should but this does not mean that you have to undertake the research yourself. It may be that the problem you have identified is shared by others in your hospital/community area. In such instances a larger project may be appropriate. One way of addressing this matter is to find out whether the Health Authority has appointed a Research Nurse who can help/advise you.

Alternatively, you may feel that you would like to develop your knowledge and understanding of research by taking a course. A course at **Diploma** level will help you to develop/enhance the skills of critically appraising existing research. Some courses will go further and help you to develop a research protocol but will not normally require students to actually conduct projects. A course at **First Degree** level will enable you to deepen your knowledge of research. It may require students to conduct a small scale project. A course at **Master's** level or above will involve you in undertaking a substantial project. This will be backed up with indepth teaching about research.

iii) It's linked to my staff development/IPR"

If such targets are being set by your manager there is a need to clarify, preferably in writing, a number of points in relation to the **cost of** the project.

Research is not without costs. Even a small scale project will involve literature searching, sending away for articles, (for which many libraries charge a fee), phone calls, typing/word processing, equipment (eg. tape recorder for interviewing), postage, travel, all of which cost money.

Who is going to pay these costs?

If your manager wants you to undertake a project, you need to raise this issue at the beginning. Obviously, at this stage neither you nor your manager will be able to discuss specific sums of money but clarifying this issue, at least in principal, is important unless you intend to meet all the costs yourself regardless of the amount.

When you have planned the method section of your protocol (Chapters 1 and 4) you will be able to calculate the specific costs involved in the project. This calculation should include:

1) **items for which there will be a charge** eg. telephone calls, postage, typing, purchase of equipment. The nature of these will arise from the methods you have selected. You may not be able to give an exact cost for some items such as telephone calls but it should be possible to estimate the approximate sum involved.

2) **your time.** How much are you paid per hour? Your time is probably the most expensive resource for the project. When are you going to undertake this work? To be expected to do so entirely in your own time could be unreasonable. Consider negotiating a regular amount of time each week to devote to the project. In doing this you will need to estimate the total

amount of time you will need to complete the work. Your estimate should include time for:

- literature searching, sending away for articles **and** having to wait for them to arrive
- reading which is very time consuming
- developing and piloting data collection tools
- collecting data - including travel, phone calls, letters etc
- transcribing/collating data - a taped interview will have to be transcribed so that it can be read. An interview of one hour could take more than four hours to transcribe. Questionnaires will have to be collated and analysed. The amount of time for this will vary but each one may take up to two hours.
- analysing data
- writing the final report
- it may also be necessary to include the cost of a replacement for you whilst you are undertaking the project but this may not apply in all instances.

Research takes time. The results are unlikely to be available after just a couple of weeks and it is probably wiser if you are also learning research skills, to slightly overestimate the amount of time required.

If your manager cannot fund the project there may be the possibility of obtaining funding from other sources. The Health Authority may have trust funds which can be used for this purpose (ask your manager). Alternatively, the usual practice is for you to approach outside agencies for financial assistance. The following publications may be of some help. Please try not to feel put off by the word "charity". For many people this word is laden with value judgements or feelings of being beholden in some way to others. In the context of undertaking research this should not be the case. Part of the function of the organisations listed below is to fund research activities on the basis that whilst they are expensive, they may yield valuable new insights into issues concerning health, illness, treatment and care and thus ultimately be of benefit to patients and their families.

Research appreciation

The Association of Medical Research Charities Handbook
Available from:
> The Association of Medical Research Charities
> Tavistock House South
> Tavistock Square
> London WC1H 9LG

The book lists a large number of charitable organisations which will donate money to research activities. It gives details of each organisation, the types of award each will make, their individual research interests plus other information.

Norton M (1991) "A Guide to Company Giving" Directory of Social Change

This gives the names and addresses of companies which donate money for research projects; their policies about doing so; who is eligible to apply and at what time of year they should do so; who to approach within the organisation.

Fitzherbert L and Eastwood M (1988) "The Educational Grants Directory" Directory of Social Change (7)

A similar publication to that of Norton (above). This book gives the names and addresses of trusts and other organisations which offer financial support for children and students in need; details of who is eligible to apply and who to contact. If you are embarking on a course of study, this book may be especially helpful.

Directory of Nursing Charities; Queen's Nursing Institute (1993); Directory of Nursing Charities; QNI London

When you write to any organisation about funding remember to state who you are and what you are proposing to research. Ask if this is the sort of work they would consider funding and whether they might be prepared to give financial support to this particular project. State clearly how much money you are looking for and try to ensure that the figure is as realistic as possible. If you are successful in obtaining funds, you are unlikely to create a favourable impression if you have to go back and ask for more or worse still the project has to be abandoned because of insufficient funds. **Be brief.** One short paragraph is more likely to achieve a response than a lengthy letter.

Conclusion

Embarking on a research project involves sorting out a number of different issues some of which may be difficult or unpleasant. It is worth taking the time to sort out where the money will come from, when you are going to have time to do the work and so on as well as developing your knowledge of research before you begin as this can only contribute positively to the success of the study. When you have sorted out these issues the rest of this book will help you to go ahead.

References

Association of Medical Research Charities Handbook. The Association of Medical Research Charities, Tavistock House South, Tavistock Square, London WC1H 9LG.

Fitzherbert L and Eastwood M (1988). *The Educational Grants Directory*, Directory of Social Change, London.

Lancet editorial (1983). *Lancet*, **8337**, 1311.

Medawar P (1967). *The Art of the Soluble*, Methuen, London.

Norton M (1991). *A guide to company giving*, Directory of Social Change, London.

Queens Nursing Institute (1993). Directory of Nuring Charities, QNI London

Walsh M and Ford P (1989). *Nursing Rituals: Research and Rational Action*, Heinemann Nursing, Oxford

Winfield U (1986). Too close a shave, *Nursing Times*, **82** (10), 64–8.

Chapter 3

How Do You Find Out?

Introduction

At the end of this chapter you will be able to:

i) conduct a literature search
ii) develop skills in critically appraising literature
iii) write a literaure review.

Why is a literature review necessary?

A comprehensive review based on a systematice search will enable you to develop insight into the subject area as a whole. You will be able to determine what research has already been undertaken with regard to the subject you wish to study, what the findings are to date, who are the principal researchers in the field and most importantly the aspects of the topic which have not so far been investigated.

Conducting a literature search

First the reality. No library will have a file marked X specifically about the topic you want to research unless you are very lucky indeed! Information is stored in libraries in a variety of different ways and when you begin your search you will have no way of knowing about the best places to look. It is like trying to unlock a safe. You need to try as many combinations as possible. There are three keys to a successful literature search. Gain access to a library, know what you are looking for and get the library staff to help you.

Research appreciation

Gaining access to a library

This will depend largely on local arrangements. In some instances you may have access to

a) The College of Nursing Library. A good College of Nursing library should have a wide range of nursing/medical journals as well as books. It will probably stock publications such as Nursing Research Abstracts and the Bibliography of Nursing Research. However few colleges can afford to allow qualified staff to borrow books but you may able to use the library for reference. Ask the librarian in the college about this.

b) Some Health Authorities have arrangements with local centres of higher education and this enables the qualified staff to have access to a University library. The best person to ask about this is probably your own senior manager.

c) All Health Authorities will have a District Information Service. Ask your manager who your District Information Officer is. They should be able to provide you with data about the population within the Authority's boundaries. They should also have access to papers and reports published by the Department of Health. The Community Health Council may also have information or may have compiled their own reports.

d) If you are a member of certain professional organisations such as the Royal College of Nursing, the organisation may have a library service which you can access but only as a member.

e) Special interest groups such as the National Association of Theatre Nurses may have additional sources of information or be able to make suggestions.

STEP SIX

IDENTIFYING KEY WORDS OR PHRASES

TIME REQUIRED: APPROXIMATELY 15-20 MINUTES.

Know what you are looking for

Look back at the brainstorming you have done. In the previous stage you have ended up with a list of items directly relevant to the subject to be researched. In the example given these were:

- Do we need to clean?
- What should beds be cleaned with?
- Is a quick wipe with soap and a wet paper towel enough?
- Is special cleaning needed if a patient has had certain conditions/infections?
- What are the costs involved in cleaning beds?
- Empty beds fill up quickly.
- Should beds be cleaned regularly even if a patient does not go home?
- Can patients catch infections from beds?

In examining this list, try to identify words or phrases which you could look up in the various sources of information which libraries have to offer. These words or phrases will, you hope, be listed in abstracts or indexes of research or in databases. Thus examples from the above list might include:

- bed cleaning
- cleaning - frequency of
- beds and infection control
- beds and cross infection
- cleaning costs
- cleaning and materials

Research appreciation

Try to generate as many of these words and phrases as you can. At this stage in the research it is impossible to know which will prove to be successful and yield the most information. Make a list of these words and phrases and always take them with you to the library. As your search progesses you will be able to cross off those which are not successful and perhaps add new ones.

Getting the librarian to help you

Libraries are essentially sources of information and one of the functions of librarians is to assist readers in finding the information they need. The librarian is there to help you but can only do so if you can present a clear idea of what you want – hence the first use for your list of key words.

Sources of information in libraries

Abstracts

These are summaries of published articles. Nursing Research Abstracts for example are published quarterly by the Department of Health and will give you summaries of a wide range of research articles usually under subject headings. Dissertation Abstracts International will give a similar summary of doctoral dissertations.

Bibliographies

These are lists of printed documents arranged in such a way that they can be easily traced. Examples include British National Biblography which is based on books received by the British Library, Books in Print, Books now Out of Print and Nursing Bibliography which is published by the Royal College of Nursing. This particular publication lists research reports alphabetically by subject heading and also has an author index.

Indexes

Most journals will publish an index of their contents, usually on an annual basis. The style of the index may vary with some using authors' names as a basis and others using subject headings. Other forms of index, such as the Index to Theses Accepted for Higher

Degrees by the Universities of Great Britain and Ireland and the Council for National and Academic Awards will help you to trace specific items of research but will not give any abstracts.

Citation Index

This is a specialised type of index consisting of a citation index and a source index both of which are arranged alphabetically. The use of the index depends on knowing the name of an author of a work relevant to the subject being researched. The user looks up the name of the author in the citation index. If other writers have referred to the author, these references will be listed and details can be traced in the source index.

The advantage of this type of index is that if you have details of one article you can link it with others published later. An example of this type of index is the Cumulated Index Medicus which is an accumulation of the monthly issues of Index Medicus. It is a very comprehensive index of publications in the field of medicine and related disciplines.

Current Awareness Library Bulletins

Many libraries produce their own indexes based on subjects of particular interest to their readers. Some will give details of books as well as journal articles. From the researcher's point of view these small scale indexes are more likely to be up to date but the quality depends heavily on the range of journals etc stocked by the library concerned.

Library Catalogue

This will give information about the documents held in the library. Some libraries actually publish their catalogues.

Conference Proceedings

Tracing conference proceedings can be difficult. Not all conference papers are published and even if they are they may not be published in full; published long after the conference; published separately.

Dictionaries For Special Use

These include glossaries of terms; quotations; subjects such as medicine or nursing; thesauri which classify words of similar meaning; biographical details eg *Who's Who*; and geographical information eg. *Gazetteers*. Included in this group are **directories** such as *Kelly's Directory* which can be used to trace the addresses of companies. Generally researchers do not report on their work until they have completed it but there are some directories which may indicate individuals' research interests or give an outline of their current work. An example is *THE BEST DIRECTORY*. **Electoral rolls** can also be used to trace private residents.

Monographs

These are short publications on specific subjects. The research reports published by the Royal College of Nursing are examples of these eg Gott M (1984) *Learning Nursing: a study of the effectiveness and relevance of teaching provided during student nurse introductory course.*

Yearbooks

This is a term used to cover a variety of reference books published annually. Examples include: *Writers' & Artists' Yearbook; Whitaker's Almanack*; and the *British Standards Yearbook*.

Newspapers

These are a valuable source of information especially if you are conducting historical research. Older papers are likely to be stored on microfilm. Some may be difficult to trace as the majority of newspapers are not indexed and the researcher has therefore to sift through back copies to trace the required material.

Government Papers

These include the reports of Parliamentary debates known as *Hansard*; reports from committees such as House of Lords, Priorities in Medical Research: Report of the select Committee on Science and Technology; consultative papers; policy papers. There are large numbers of government papers many of which receive very little publicity. The best place to start in trying to trace government papers is the the HMSO serials catalogues. HMSO is the main publisher for government papers and the catalogues are cumulative so that it is possible to trace older papers.

Censuses and Surveys

These will give statistical information about a wide range of topics. An example is *Social Trends* which gives information about the UK based on census data and surveys on a wide range of issues such as housing, the envirnoment, employment etc. It is updated annually.

Patents and Standards

Patent specifications are published by the British Patent Office and give information about inventions and their owners. Patents can provide a great deal of technical information but not every library will stock information of this kind. To trace patents you will need to consult the British Library Science Reference Library in London or the Patent Information Network Bulletin. Standards are formulated by committees of experts to regulate manufactured goods of safety, size, quality etc. All British standards can be found in the British Standards Yearbook.

Finding what you want

This is where you will need the help of the librarian. Browsing along the shelves may be very interesting but it is unlikely to yield much in the way of results. Searching for information must be systematic and thorough if it is to be of any use in your project. There are two ways of doing this:

Manual searching involves looking through the abstracts and other sources manually beginning with the most recent editions and working backwards. You will need to use your key words and phrases to do this. It is useful to keep a record of what you have searched through as it is unlikely that you will be able to complete a search quickly. One way of doing this is to list your key words/phrases (Table 3.1) and the publications you are searching through and tick them off as you go.

Research appreciation

Table 3.1: Recording your search

KEY WORDS	NURSING RESEARCH ABSTRACTS					
	1992	1991	1990	1989	1988	1987
Bed cleaning	/	/	/			
Cleaning – frequency of	/	/	/			
Beds and infection control	/	/				
Beds and cross-infection	/	/				
Cleaning costs	/	/				
Cleaning and materials	/	/				

When you have found items which seem useful you will need to note down the full reference.

The advantages of this type of search is that you may come across the unexpected but on the whole it is very time consuming and tiring.

Computer searching involves searching through published material on a compact disc. Many libraries now have this CD ROM facility. The data stored on the disc is collated from a variety of published sources. Larger systems such as Medline will have a compact disc for each year. The same principle applies as with manual searches. Begin with the most recent disc, present your key words to the computer which is able to search through its' database for appropriate material. Details of this with abstracts are then shown on a screen and a printout of the reference can be obtained. Keep a list of your key words/phrases and tick them off as you complete your search on each disc.

The main advantage of this type of search is that it is very fast. In one hour it is possible to trace quite a lot of material. However, a machine can only do what it is told to do and consequently the success of the search depends heavily on the appropriateness of the key words/phrases. Moreover it is possible that not everything published is actually on the compact discs and it may therefore be possible to miss useful information.

How far back should I search?"

There is no hard and fast rule but it is probably wise to start with the current year and work backwards for about five years. This approach is likely to yield the most up to date material. You can then go back another five years if you wish and so on.

"What if I don't find anything?"

There are a number of possibilities. First of all have you searched enough? There may not have been anything published within the last five years. You may need to try further back. If you are still unsuccessful you may need to consider developing some additional key words/phrases just in case your search is too narrowly focused. An additional strategy is to look outside you own field of expertise. In the example given:

- bed cleaning
- cleaning - frequency of
- beds and infection control
- beds and cross infection
- cleaning costs
- cleaning and materials

It might be helpful to search not only nursing literature but also that on microbiology, infection control and hotel services. Finally you may have to accept that little or nothing has been published on your topic. **This is not a reason to abandon your research!** On the contrary it indicates that this is an under-researched field which needs attention.

"I've got so much!

Certain aspects of nursing are extremely popular with researchers. Topics like the Nursing Process have generated a vast quantity of articles and books. In this instance you may need to consider having very specific key words/phrases and searching two years at a time rather than five.

Research appreciation

"When should I stop?"

When you feel you have a reasonable number of items to read. There is no set rule about this but about twenty items should be enough to get started especially as you will probably get more references from them. Some searches will of course not yield as many items as this whilst others may produce a lot more. The important thing to remember is that once you have obtained the references you then have to find the articles or books on the library shelves or send away for them through the inter-library loan system. This can take quite a lot of time. You then have to sit down and read all the material which again takes time so the sooner you get started the better. You can always repeat or extend the search as your reading progresses.

STEP SEVEN

RECORDING AND TAKING NOTES

KEEP A RECORD OF EVERYTHING YOU READ - EVEN IF IT IS NO OF USE

Constructing the literature review

You will very quickly find that you are swamped with information and it is easy at this stage to feel overwhelmed by it all. Also you may forget what you have read and this can waste a lot of time. This is a strategy which may help. You will need two card index boxes, some dividers and some index cards.

How do you find out?

BOX ONE

Write a card for each item you read.
If it is a book record the following:
- ¤ *Surname: initials: year of publication: title publisher: place of publication: ie. London, New York; edition*

Add a few brief notes about what you have read.
If it is an article in a journal record the following:
- ¤ *Surname: initials: year of publication: title (of the article): title of the journal: part number: volume number: page numbers of the article*

Add a few brief notes about what you have read.

File all the cards in alphabetical order in the box. Try to establish the habit of completing a card every time you read something even if the book/article is not much help. The advantage of this system is that it enables you to keep a record of everything you read; identify the major writers in the field and keep track of when material has been published.

Research appreciation

BOX TWO

As your reading progresses try to identify themes which emerge from the literature. As an example, a review of the literature on bed cleaning nursing might yield the following themes:
- bed cleaning materials
- bad cleaning costs
- bed cleaning and infectious diseases
- bed cleaning and nurse training
- history of bed cleaning
- DOH recommendations on bed cleaning
- hospital policies

Write a card for each item you read.
Record the following
- *Surname: year of publication: title*

Brief notes about the book/article.
File the cards under the different themes or topics you have identified.

The advantage of this system is that it enables you to group material together and identify issues which are important. It also helps in structuring your writing - all the relevant references are already grouped together before you start.

STEP EIGHT

CRITICALLY APPRAISING THE LITERATURE

Don't believe everything you read in a book! As you read try to identify the strengths and weaknesses of every item you read. The following points will help.

i) **Is this research or the writer's opinion?**

Opinions are fine but they are not based on research. They may, therefore, be based not on systematic enquiry but on a range of other factors such as feelings, prejudices and personal quirks.

Consequently they cannot be applied to other situations with confidence or rigour.

ii) How clear is each stage of the research process?

The clarity of the research question, the literature review, the methodology etc should each be questioned. In particular, the way in which statistics are presented is important. As Huff (1954) argues, it is possible to present statistics in a misleading way and imply things which are, in fact, untrue.

Clarity has two dimensions — **semantic clarity** refers to the use of language; whether the terminology used is clear and accurate. Tripp-Reimer and Dougherty (1985) have criticised nursing research for:

> 'the inappropriate or inaccurate use of terms, concepts, and methods originating in other disciplines".

In addition, the terminology used must be consistent throughout. This is particularly important when looking at the work of a writer over time. Terminology used in early work on the subject must be consistent with that used in more recent publications. **Structural clarity** refers to the clarity of ideas expressed both here and now and as the writer's work develops over the years.

iii) What are the underlying influences on the writer?

In describing her model of nursing, Roy, for example, acknowledges the influence of Helson and Johnson. In a more general sense, writers may show a leaning towards explaining events from the perspective of a particular discipline eg. physiology, psychology etc which may mean that the ideas expressed need to be balanced against those offered by other sources. Finally there may be evidence of vested interest. Usually, it does not matter who has funded a research project, but a project funded by a tobacco company which states that smoking does no harm might invite some scepticism.

iv) How generalisable are the results?

The concepts of **reliability** and **validity** are important here; these terms have very specific meanings in research. Validity is the

Research appreciation

degree to which a particular research method (questionnaire, interview schedule, observation grid, etc.) measures what itsets out to achieve (Shaw and Wright, 1967). Validity has two dimensions internal and external. **Internal validity** is concerned with those factors within the project which may affect the methods chosen. A project is said to be internally valid if, within its own confines, the results are credible. In other words the tool used for data collection has provided the type of data it was designed to collect. However, for those results to be useful they must be generalisable to other settings.**External validity** is concerned with factors which limit the degree to which the results of the project can be applied to other settings. A project may have internal validity and yet not produce results which can be applied in other settings. (Cohen and Mannion, 1989; Shaw and Wright, 1967).

Reliability is the extent to which the tool yields consistent results each time it is used (Monette *et al* 1990). Just as you would expect reliable weighing scales to read the same each time you put the same weight on them, so in research a reliable tool is one that, if used repeatedly, will give similar data each time.

However, it must be pointed out that reliability and validity do not ensure accuracy. A tool can be valid (measure what it sets out to measure) and reliable (yield consistent data) but, if the questions asked are inappropriate, based on incorrect or limited information, or the groups studied has very different characteristics to the one the tool was designed for, then the findings of the project will not be accurate and generalisable.

STEP NINE

CONSTRUCTING THE LITERATURE REVIEW

If you have used the topic box outlined in step seven you will already have identified the main themes emerging from the literature. Your next step is to plan your review around these themes begining with those you consider to be the most important. Write about each theme using the literature to support your argument. For example:

> *"Wound care management has changed dramatically over the last ten years as a result of research into healing and tissues repair (Fergusson 1988). However, despite evidence of their harmful effects, hypochlorite solutions are still being used in both hospitals and the community eg for wound debridement in the treatment of leg ulcers and burns (Saunders 1989; Catlin 1992)."*

This extract shows that the writer has integrated material from different sources. You do not have to use every item you have read. Choose the most appropriate item for the points you are trying to make and present them in a logical sequence, so that the reader can see how you have used the literature and research to develop and present an argument or discussion supporting the need for your project.

You should comment on the methods researchers have used. If all previous studies have used similar methods to collect and analyse their data, you can point this out and argue the need for an alternative approach (if that is what you plan). If previous studies have all been exploratory in nature, you can use this to point out the need for more research before findings can be used on a wider scale. Similarly, if a study seems useful but you think it is too small to be generalisable you can still use it in your discussion provided you include the limitations of the project as well as the findings.

Remember to give a balanced argument ie. where the literature you have gathered shows that there are major differences in attitude, treatment etc, comment on these. You can use them to show the need for more research in this field to clarify the situation and you should describe how your project will inform the debate. Where the review shows gaps in available data and literature, you can discuss how your project might help fill in some of these gaps.

Finally, a word of caution. It is very easy to become sidetracked into presenting information you have gathered because you find it interesting and not because it provides a necessary part of the background to your study. Once you think you have completed your discussion, you need to check that you have 'set the scene' for your project and have not just given an interesting argument.

Conclusion

Finding out what has already been published about the subject you want to research requires some special skills and access to good library facilities. Searching for appropriate literature can be time consuming. It is important to read critically identifying the strengths and weaknesses of each item of literature. A good literature review should provide an overview of the research already conducted; identify gaps or limitations in the research; act as a sounding board for ideas. It will also pave the way for your choice of research method.

References

Catlin L (1992). The Use of Hypochlorite Solutions in Wound Management *Br J Nurs*, **1:5**, 226–9

Cohen L and Mannion L (1989). *Research Methods in Education, 3rd edn*, Routledge, London.

Denzin N (1989) *The Research Act, 3rd edn,* Prentice Hall, New Jersey.

Huff D (1954). *How to lie with statistics*, Republished 1973 by Pelican, London

Monette D, Sullivan T and DeJong C (1990). *Applied social research,* Holt, Rinehart and Winston, Fort Worth

Shaw M and Wright J (1967). *Scales for the measurements of attitudes,* McGraw Hill, New York

Tripp-Reimer T and Dougherty M (1985). Cross-cultural Nursing Research, *Ann Rev Nurs Res*, **3**, 77–104

Chapter 4
Whom can you ask?

You have now decided what you want to know and are collecting information about what has already been studied. As you read the literature you will gain an idea of the research methods that other researchers have used to gather data. So these next two chapters have been designed to help you decide whether or not you want to use a method that has been used before, or whether you want to try something else.

Before starting any project you need to consider two things:

1) who are you going to use as respondents in your study, and

2) what sort of information do you need to gather.

This chapter will look at the first of these two areas, by the end of this chapter you will be able to:

i) discuss the terms used when groups of people are studied

ii) describe the different groups that can be used in research

Sampling

Sampling is the name given to the process of deciding who to contact. In this process the terms **population** and **target population** are frequently used but here they do not necessarily refer to a country's total population or the number of people in a geographical location. Instead they may refer to the group of people, households, individuals etc. that the researcher is investigating, and it is from this selected group that the respondents for the study are drawn, we call the respondents **the Sample**.

If the target population is small (for instance people with a rare disease) then you may be able to contact all of them. When you are able to do this you are said to be carrying out a type of small scale **census**. However this can be both costly and time comsuming (as people may be scattered across the whole country) and usually we choose to contact only a proportion of the total group. Similarly where there is a large number of people in the group for practical reasons you would only be able to contact a small proportion. The idea is to select a sample that will behave or give the same range of responses as all the other people in the population. In other words, you try to find a group that can be said to be **representative** of the total population and therefore you can use your findings to make inferences about the whole population.

Often it is relatively easy to define the target population but gaining access to a representative sample is much more difficult and there are several standard **sampling frames** that can be used to try to overcome the problem of identifying individuals and/or specific households:

1) *The Electoral Register* provides the names of all individuals over 18 and their addresses listed in voting districts. The main drawback to this register is that it is only updated once each year and it is generally accepted that in large urban areas with mobile populations it may be up to 30% inaccurate.

2) *Government Departments* record a wide range of information which include registers of factories, schools together with the numbers of children attending, national insurance records, and unemployment. However the available lists may not be up to date (in some instances it takes 1-2 years before lists are updated) and, access to the data may be severely restricted.

3) *Private clubs and institutions* usually keep lists of members but as club officials feel a measure of responsibility for maintaining confidentiality gaining access is often difficult and time-consuming. However if the project can be seen to benefit members clubs can be very co-operative.

4 *Computer data bases* Although the government has taken considerable steps to protect individuals, it is still possible to access

some computer lists, particularly if you are working in conjunction with industry or commerce.

5) *Professional Organisations* Again as with private clubs there may be problems gaining access and projects usually have to be approved by the organisations officials, and contact may be arranged only through the organisation ie. they will contact the individual members for you.

6) *Census* The national census is conducted every 10 years. Data is usually available 1-2 years after each census. Until the 1980's a mini-census was conducted at the mid-point between each national census with the 80's being the first decade to not to have one.

7) *Residents associations* These can be useful but tend to exist in more settled areas so where there are highly mobile populations they may not exist, and it is important to remember that they may not be representative of the local population.

8) *Professional research agencies* There are some 200 organisations that offer research services and these vary in size from small local agencies to large organisations such as Gallup, MORI, RSGB. They can usually provide a service that varies from identifying the sample within the target population to designing and carrying out the actual research project.

9) *Local authority records* Such as community charge lists, these are updated annually but are still not very accurate where there are highly mobile populations.

10) *Hospital activity records* These are records of everyone admitted to hospital, together with when and to where they were discharged. They also contain information about the range of diseases and disorders treated. Physical illness, Mental illness and maternity statistics are all recorded separately so you may need to contact several different centres.

11) **GP records** These have become more useful as computerisation has occurred. You may only gain access if the GPs give permission as they have the responsibilty of guarding the data about their patients. However if they agree you can access a wide range of information including types of disease and illness, frequency of attendance, treatments used etc.

12) **Colleges of nursing** These are really just lists of members but can be extremely useful if you wish to contact nurses with particlar expertise and/or interests.

13) **Community nursing records** These records although very detailed about patients cared for by community nurses, as with GP records access may be restricted.

Sample Size

As you may have gathered, sampling is usually a matter of compromise whilst trying to ensure that the sample is as representative as possible you are constrained by the nature of the topic, the time and resources that you have available for the whole project. Obviously, the sample for a qualitative study will be smaller than that for a quantitative survey, but it is worth noting that although a sample of 400 respondents is likely to be more representative than one of 200, it is **not** twice as representative. As a rough guide many national surveys only have around 1000 respondents and the law of diminishing returns means that the extra precison gained from having a large sample may not be worth the time and effort involved.

To enable people to understand the way you have decided which people to contact there are special terms used to describe different types of groups of people. These are:

Simple Random Samples

This is a method of sample selection by which every member of the target population has an equal chance of being selected. This maximises the chance of the sample being representative of the target population and minimises the possibility of bias. For this type of sample you need an up-to-date sampling frame (list of the target population). Selection could be by making a list of the total number of individuals in the target population, putting all the numbers in a hat, then taking the numbers out of the hat until you have sufficient respondents for your project. Alternatively, you can use tables specially constructed (by computer) and called random tables.

Systematic Samples

This is probably the most commonly used method of sample selection for social surveys and works well for both small and large scale surveys. Starting with a sampling frame you randomly select the first number (or case) from a list of all possible respondents (the total sampling frame) by closing your eyes and sticking a pin in the list. This is then your starting point and the principle is based on selection of cases using a sampling ratio. For instance if you wanted a sample of 100 from a target population of 1000 your ratio would be 1:10 so, having selected your first case you would go on to select every tenth person on your list. If you reach the end of your list before you have extracted enough names you simply start from the top again treating the first name as if it were on the end of the list and continue until you have all the names you need.

It is worth noting that with this type of sample you have to check that your original sampling frame (list) does not have particular categories of household or occupation grouped together as this could result in a biased sample that either completely misses out one or more categories within your target population, or alternatively consists entirely of one particular one. For example if you wanted to contact people on different wards, if all have the same number of staff, then if you contact every 10th nurse (on each ward) you might find that all your respondents are from similar grades so you wouldn't have a true overview of all perspectives.

Stratified Samples

As the name suggests with this type of sample the target population is divided into layers or strata. Usually the division used is one that relates to your research, and you then select your sample from within the chosen strata. This type of sample is used when instead of studying the whole population you wish to look at particular groups within the population. For instance you may wish to compare the attitudes that different age groups have concerning a specific issue. Your layers or strata would in this case be the different age bands. Alternatively you may select a particular occupational group such as teachers, nurses etc.

Within your chosen strata you can either select proportionately according to the characteristics of the group and/or to preserve the overall balance of your sample or, you can select disproportionately using specific criteria. You might decide that one particular group within your strata is a **critical case**. This is a group that for some reason is either different from the rest of the possible respondents or, has particular relevance for the issue that you are studying. For example you may only want to select head teachers rather than a sample of all teachers.

Cluster Samples

A cluster sample is one where the target population is grouped together to form clusters. There are all kinds of ready made clusters such as clubs, schools, factories, hospitals, streets, villages, towns or types of housing. Cluster samples tend to show a degree of conformity because the reason for the cluster existing may well be an influencing factor, for example occupation (if the cluster is a factory or other institution) or type and cost of housing (if the cluster is based on a street, village or town). As with stratified sampling it may be that a particular cluster is seen as very important or as a critical case and so is studied in its entirety. Alternatively a systematic or random sample may be drawn from within one or more clusters.

The main advantages of using cluster samples are that you do not need a sampling frame for the whole population and contacting the chosen cluster is usually quicker and cheaper than methods which involve the total population. However it is important to realise that this method of sampling can lead to a large percentage of the total population being excluded from study.

Quota Samples

This is a popular method of sample selection for market researchers, it is based on an interviewer selecting respondents to meet previously decided criteria. These criteria are usually based on variables such as age, sex, occupation and class and the interviewer has to select a given number of people for each particular set of criteria. For ease, quota samples are often set out in tabloid form with each cell (square) indicating how many people should be interviewed (Table 4.1).

Table 4.1: Example of a quota sample table for female respondents

	Social Class					
Age	I	II	IIIn	IIIm	IV	V
20–29	10	10	10	10	10	10
30–39	10	10	10	10	10	10
40–49	10	10	10	10	10	10
50–59	8	8	8	8	8	8
60–69	6	6	6	6	6	6

Total number in sample = 164
Note: The different numbers in the cells are based on the age distribution within the target population. To have interviewed the same number in each category would have meant the sample was not repesentative of the target population.

The main advantages of this method are that it is cheap, simple to use and quick. If the respondent does not fit the criteria (this is ascertained at the start of the interview) they are rejected and time is not wasted on interviews that cannot be used. However the disadvantages are that the interviewer actually selects the sample so their own bias and prejudice may affect the choice of respondents. In addition it can take a long time to find the the correct number of respondents in each category and complete the sample.

Voluntary Samples

As the name suggests these are self-selected samples, people participate if they want to. Forms are often left out on counters or desks where interested individuals can pick them up and complete them if they choose. Postal surveys can use this type of sample as they can sent out their questionnaires through the post and only if the recipient chooses to join in, will the form be returned. Obviously this means that there is no way that you can ensure that the sample is representative, particularly as it is now thought that people who choose to participate in studies may share certain characteristics. However it may still be a valid method to use for exploratory studies or to try to see which issues could be expanded and studied in detail.

Snowball Samples

Snowball samples are used when the target population is not easy to contact and/ or even if you can find them access may be limited. The people who fit into this category are minority groups, those that are being discriminated against, or those that do not wish other people to know that they belong to a particular sect or group. Quite simply the method of selection is by word of mouth or by by letter, you contact a few people from within the target population and then ask them if they can suggest other people to participate in your project.

Convenience Samples

As the name suggests, this type of sample is drawn from groups available to the researcher. This approach is popular when it is difficult (or very expensive) to develop a complete sampling frame. For example, suppose you wished to contact single fathers with children aged 5–11 years, you would probably find it extremely difficult to compile a frame of all suitable single fathers. Therefore, you might contact local schools and, through them, the required number of respondents. The biggest drawback to this approach sampling is that, as with voluntary and snowball sampling, the respondents may well not be representative of the population as a whole and there is, therefore, limited generalisability.

Non-response

It doesn't matter how carefully you select your sample, bias and non- representative results can still arise because of non or limited response. People may be out when you call, your list may be out of date, not everyone is willing to participate, postal questionnaires may get lost or not be completed particularly where there is a literacy or language problem.

With postal questionnaires an initial response of 50% is not unusual but this may increase if a reminder letter is sent.

National interview surveys rarely manage to achieve above 80% response because of time constraints and you should aim to minimise non-response as much as you can, but accept that you are unlikely to achieve 100%. Using extra respondents may increase the representativeness of your study but as non participation is not random it may not remove any bias.

Sampling Theory

There is a considerable amount of statisical and mathematical theory which is designed to assess the degree of error and representativeness of a sample. This is based on the assumption that samples are randomly selected, the size of the sample, the size of the population and any known population characteristics.

You do not need to learn all these theories to carry out research, instead a basic understanding of what some of the terms mean and when it is relevant to use particular tests is usually enough, provided that you remember that the findings of sample surveys are only **estimates** or **approximations** of population characteristics.

Two frequently used terms are:

1) significance level

2) confidence interval

1) **Significance level** The findings of social surveys are often presented as applying at particular levels of significance. This refers to the liklihood of your finding occuring by chance. Usually we say that if a finding is likely to occur by **chance** five times or less in every 100 times we would accept the findings as significant, and

Research appreciation

we call this the **5%** significance level. This is often written as 0.05 not 5%.

0.05 level of significance means that as your result would only occur by chance **5 times in 100,** for **95 times in 100** it would be a reliable estimate for the population that you are studying.

0.01 level of significance means that as your result would only occur by chance **1 time in 100,** for **99 times in 100** it would be a reliable estimate for the population you are studying.

0.001 level of significance means that as your result would only occur by chance **1 time in 1000,** for **99 times in 1000** the finding would be a reliable estimate for the population you are studying.

The smaller the level of significance used, the more likely your finding is to be significant. So 0.001 (0.1%) is a stronger measure of significance than the 0.05 (5%).

2) Confidence Interval

This is an attempt to put a precise mathematical limit to the possible error in a project. It is often used in opinion polls and written as follows:

Should income tax be abolished?

Yes 39%: No 42%: Confidence interval ± 3% at 5% level of significance

This means that 95 times in 100 the proportion of people who want the tax abolished might be anywhere between 39% plus or minus 3%, ie. between 36% and 42% Similarly those who do not want the tax abolished are between 39% and 45%

The figures above suggest that less people want the tax abolished, but, as the confidence interval shows, in reality the figures could be the other way around. It is always worth checking the figures to see if this could happen when confidence intervals are used. If the figures can be reversed, then you would be cautious about accepting the findings as representative.

The ±3 is worked out statistically based on standard deviations (see chapter 7) and is used as a measure of the error in the representativeness of the sample. It recognises that your sampling procedure may not have give as accurate a reflection of the population as would be ideal, and hency by saying your fingings come within a range of 6 (±3) you have recognised the limitation of your study.

References

Monette D R and Sullivan T J and DeJong C R (1990). *Applied social research 2nd edn*, Holt, Reinhart and Winston, USA

Phillips D R (1981). *Do-it-yourself social surveys: A handbook for beginners,* Polytechnic of North London, London.

Chapter 5
Will People Agree to Take Part?

Introduction

At the end of this chapter you will be able to:

i) begin to address some of the common ethical issues in the design and conduct of research.

In addition to planning what you are going to do by way of sampling and data collection you also need to consider whether the method you have chosen and the manner in which you plan to apply it are acceptable both to the subjects and society generally.

What are ethics?

Ethics have their origin in the values, attitudes and beliefs which form the basis of every society. They are concerned with what people believe **ought** to happen. They are rarely explicit and consequently are difficult to pin down. Moreover society is constantly changing and different groups within it may hold conflicting values, attitudes and beliefs. The clarification of ethics and what is ethical therefore requires constant debate.

According to Denzin (1989) *"It is impossible not to take ethical and value stances in the process of research"* since almost everything the researcher does involves making value laden decisions. Spradley (1980) argues that researchers have a responsibility to safeguard the rights, interests and sensitivities of their research subjects. How then can the researcher achieve this? Seedhouse (1988) provides a useful framework for ethics in health care which he sees as being concerned with:

autonomy – the capability and capacity of the individual to think and act as an independent person.

justice – which is concerned with respecting persons equally and seeking to meet the needs of individuals ensuring that these needs are not denied or obscured by the wants of society.

beneficence – which is the capacity to do good to others and for oneself.

minimising harm – which is concerned with doing the least harm to an individual.

Ethical issues in research design

All research involving human beings has ethical dimensions and should therefore be scrutinised for its potential to harm people and the ways in which that harm may be prevented or minimised. Specific areas of concern are:

i) access to potential subjects

Whether you wish to research patients in a hospital/community setting, staff, your colleagues or your students you need to consider whose permission you need before you may approach them. In other words, who is responsible for safeguarding the interests of these individuals with regard to research activities (**beneficence and minimising harm**)? The researcher must recognise that access to potential subjects is a priviledge and not a right. You must, therefore, consider from whom permission for access must be sought, the Data Protection Act and the rights to privacy of the individual.

Applying for access usually involves a chain of personnel. To begin with, the researcher must find out which committee in the Health Authority or Trust deals with reviewing the research proposals and conferring approval from an ethical perspective. All proposed research must be presented to the committee before it begins. In addition there may be other committees within the organisation or even outside, which also need to be approached for access eg.the Local Education Authority for studies to be undertaken in schools.

Having obtained permission from the committee, it will then be neccesary to seek the permission of consultants, general practitioners and managers in specific departments, each of whom is **autonomous** in this form of decision-making and may grant or refuse access as they see fit.

ii) the nature of participation

The concepts of justice and minimising harm must be considered within the context of the research methods to be used. Some methods may involve invasive procedures such as taking blood; surgery such as taking biopsies; testing out new drugs/treatments all of which are potentially harmful to the participants. The researcher has a responsibility to demonstrate to those who control access to potential subjects that s/he is competent to carry out the procedures involved and is trustworthy in handling confidential information, both written and verbal, about individuals that they may not wish others to know.

iii) recruitment

Within this context it is important to consider how you will set about approaching individual people who might be suitable to take part in the research and telling them who you are; what the research is about; what their participation would involve and possible side effects or consequences that might ensue (**justice, beneficence and minimising harm**). Information both verbal and in writing should be presented to each individual so that they can make an informed decision about whether to participate (**autonomy**). The researcher must recognise that research is separate from other activities. It is not an essential to the potential subject in the same way as treatment or conditions of employment.

The information you provide should, therefore, make clear that this is a research project and state who the researcher is, the purpose of the research and what the participants are required to do. The individual must be assured of confidentiality and also assured that s/he is not obliged to take part in the research. (Fig. 5.1)

> **Fig. 5.1: INFORMATION SHEET:**
> **a comparative study of two differing wound care procedures**
>
> I am a nurse specialising in Accident and Emergency care at this hospital. I am undertaking a course at..............................(name of college) and as a part of my studies I am trying to find out about the best method of applying dressings.
>
> The purpose of this letter is to ask whether you would be able to help in this. If you agree, you will be assigned to one of two groups of patients who visit the department for their dressings to be changed. Each group will have their dressings changed using a different method. On your last visit you will be interviewed briefly about your dressings. This interview will take about 15 minutes.
>
> All information about you and your wound and any information you give will be treated in the strictest confidence and used only for the purposes of the study. You do not have to take part if you do not wish to do so and you may withdraw at any time if you wish without affecting your treatment or care.
>
> If you do feel able to take part please sign the consent form below and keep the second copy of this letter for your own reference.
>
>   Thank you.
>
>   Yours sincerely,
>   (nurse's name)

iii) consent

The concepts of justice and autonomy in obtaining the consent of potential participants are important here. Consent will be invalidated if duress is used. Consent must only be obtained after the individual has been given a verbal and written explanation of the research and had the opportuniity to ask questions about his/her involvement. Each individual should be asked to sign a consent form which must make clear that they are free to withdraw at any time and that taking part in the research will in no way affect their current treatment/care/employment. (Fig. 5.2)

There is a belief, widespread in nursing, that consent is only required if the research involves patients. This is **not** the case.

> **Fig. 5.2 CONSENT FORM:**
> **a comparative study of two differing wound care procedures**
> I ....(patient's name) of
> ....(address) agree to
> take part in the above study which has been explained to me by
> ....(name). I understand that this will
> not affect my treatment in any way and that I may withdraw at
> any time.
>   Signed . . . .
>   Date . . . .

Studies which involve staff, relatives or other groups still require consent from each individual. Researching colleagues or subordinates can be a cause of insecurity for the individuals concerned. *"Are we being spied on? What will happen to the information? Will we be disciplined if we say the wrong thing?"* These are legitimate concerns on the part of staff who are at work primarily to earn a living. Staff must therefore be seen in the same light as other potential subjects with regard to the design and conduct of research.

Consent from special groups

There are certain types of research which require different approaches to those outlined above. For example, it may not be possible to obtain written consent from individuals with literacy problems. In such circumstances it is neccessary to seek advice form an experienced researcher.

In addition there are certain groups in society which require greater protection than others in matters to do with research. Ideally members of these groups should not be included in research studies but there may be times when it is essential that they are.

a) Children. The researcher must obtain consent from at least one parent or guardian in writing. In addition the child must be given information which is commensurate with his/her age and understanding. A child is deemed capable of giving assent, which means their agreement even if they cannot in legal terms give their consent. The child's assent must be obtained without duress from either the researcher or other parties.

b) People with mental health problems and people with learning difficulties The researcher will need to seek advice from specialists in these fields before embarking on any research.

c) Prisoners and young offenders are generally regarded as a special category in relation to research activities and the researcher must seek specialist advice if wishing to study this group.

iv) confidentiality.

The concepts of justice and minimising harm apply here in consideration of the protection of those who agree to participate in the research. Subjects must be assured in writing that the information they give will be used only for the purposes of the research (Fig. 5.1) and that they will not be indentified personally in any way either through name, address, place of work, hospital, GP, Health Authority or any other means.

Ethical issues in the conduct of research

The collection and analysis of data involves a range of ethical decision making. Generally concerns must centre on the honesty and integrity of the researcher. The researcher is expected to follow the procedures set out in the protocol once it has approved by the committees and managers concerned. Deviations from the agreed protocol must be renegotiated. Data must be presented honestly even if it conflicts with the researcher's deeply cherished beliefs.

Conclusion

The research process involves ethical issues at every stage. The design of the protocol must ensure that potential subjects will not be harmed by taking part in the study.

References

Denzin N (1989). *The Research Act* 3rd edn, Prentice Hall, New Jersey

Seedhouse D (1988). *Ethics: the heart of health care.* John Wiley and Sons, Chichester

Spradley J (1980). *Participant observation*, Holt Rinehart Winston, New York

Useful Reading

Bainham A (1990). Children - the new law, The Children's Act 1989, Family Law, Bristol

Beauchamp T and Childress J (1988). *Principles of biomedical ethics. 3rd edn.* Oxford University Press, New York.

Department of Health (1991) *Local research ethics committees.* HMSO

Gillon R (1985) *Philosophical medical ethics.* John Wiley and Sons.

Meyers D (1990). *The human body and the law*, Edinburgh University Press, Edinburgh

Royal College of Physicians (1990) *Guidelines on the practice of ethics committees in medical research involving human subjects. 2nd. edn.* Royal College of Physicians, London

Royal College of Physicians (1990) *Research involving patients.* Royal College of Physicians, London

Royal College of Physicians (1986) *Research on health volunteers.* Royal College of Physicians, London

Chapter 6
What can you find out

Now that you know what type and size of sample you are going to use you can move on to decide what sort of information you need to collect. This chapter will discuss the different methods giving some of the advantages and disadvantages of each one.

By the end of this chapter you should be able to:

i) describe the main methods of data collection

ii) design and administer a questionnaire

iii) plan and conduct an interview

iv) use observation techniques to gather information

Methods of Data Collection

Surveys

Surveys are still one of the most popular methods of collecting data. They are a means of collecting information by using questionnaires or structured interviews. Questionnaires are usually used if a large samples chosen because the advantage of this method is that of cost effectiveness. There are several stages to a survey (Hoinville *et al* 1978) and we have chosen to illustrate them as they do, through the description of a postal survey. Fig 6.1 shows the different stages and, as you can see, once the questionnaire has been designed, it is relatively easy to administer and the collection of the data is straight forward.

It is important to know that with this type of research many of the potential respondents will not complete and return the questionnaire, so a 50% response is good (Oppenheim 1990). Postal reminders are essential if you wish to increase your response rate,

Research appreciation

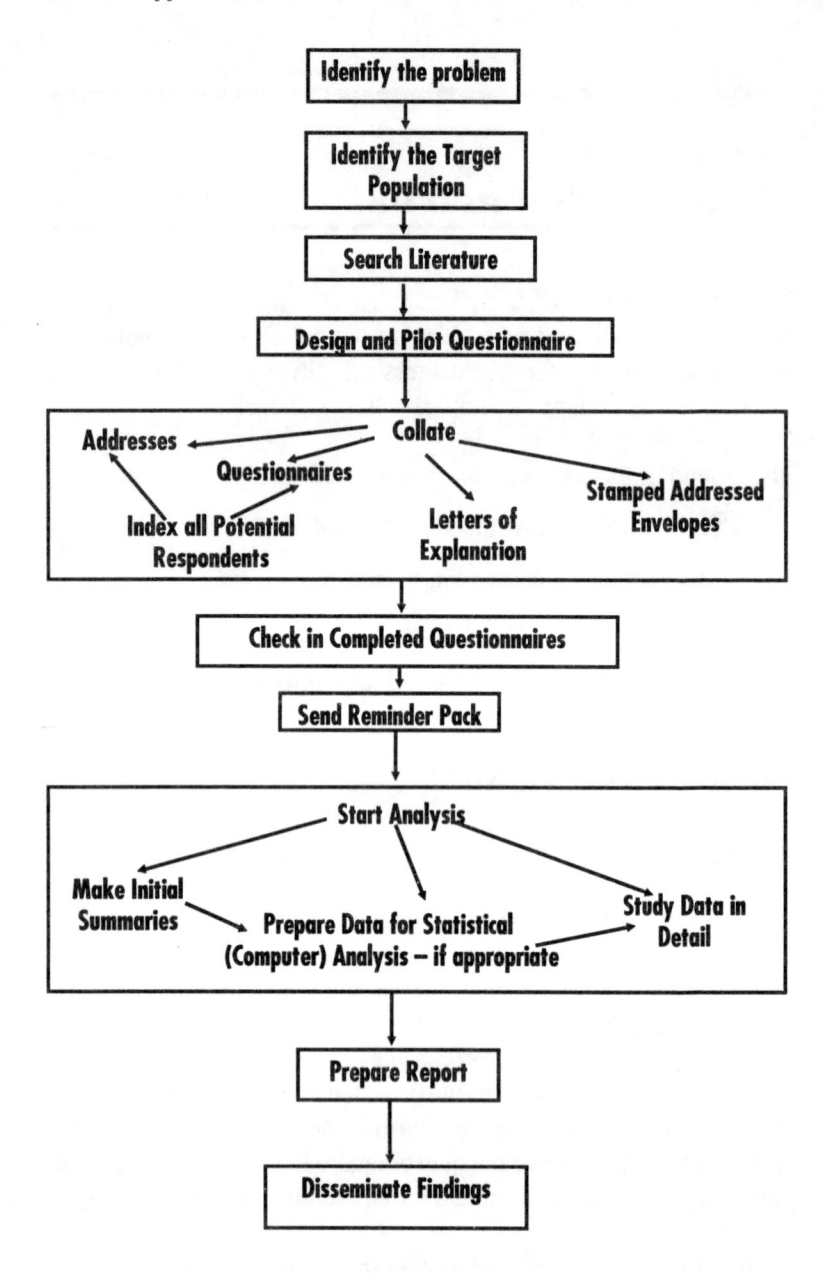

Figure 6.1: The stages in a survey

and you should always include another copy of the questionnaire as it is inevitable that some will be misplaced.

The importance of a well designed questionnaire cannot be overestimated because it provides the link between the researcher and respondents (Moser and Kalton 1978). You are more likely to have a good response if your questionnaire is well laid out and easy to complete.

Whatever the subject, size or length of the questionnaire, you need to follow certain basic rules. Construction can be divided into two parts:

1) the overall layout and content
2) the wording and order of the questions.

Overall layout and content

Ideally there should be an accompanying letter explaining what the project is about and ensuring the respondents of the confidentiality of their responses. It also encourages participation if you can say when and where the findings will be available. As well as including the letter of explanation one sentence at the start of the questionnaire summarising the project is helpful because the original letter may easily become lost and if the respondent cannot remember what the project is about they may decide it's not worth completing the questionnaire.

It is essential that when your questionnaire is complete it is attractive to look at and easy to read. A questionnaire that looks complicated or messy will discourage potential respondents and may well increase your no-response rate.

A good test of your final layout is to ask someone not connected with the project to read and complete the form and then give you their comments.

Before deciding the actual questions make a list of the topic areas that you wish to cover. Once you have done this, decide which subjects can link with each other and then go through the list deciding just how important each topic is. Be ruthless. Leave out anything that is not essential. If you don't compile a list but go straight into designing the questions you may well find that when you come to analyse your data you either have quantities of data that you cannot use, or you have not covered all the important issues in sufficient detail.

At this stage it may be worth doing a small amount of preliminary work to clarify which of your topic areas are going to provide the most useful data. There are different ways of doing this. You can discuss the subject with 'experts', you could conduct a few general discussions with people from your target group or you could recheck previous research reports looking, particularly, at the data gathered. If the issue is of general interest, media programmes and articles may provide additional insights.

The final length of your questionnaire will be governed by the subject that you have chosen to study. The preliminary work and your literature search will have shown which areas are essential, but generally speaking the shorter the questionnaire the better. Unless you are studying a subject that your target group will find absorbing (eg sportsmen discussing their particular sport) a questionnaire that is long and rambling will discourage all but the most determined. It is not unusual for respondents presented a very lengthy questionnaire to give up and either send back a half completed form or not send it back at all.

As a general rule, a questionnaire that is to be administered and/or completed by an interviewer can be longer than one that is self-completed as the interviewer can encourage the respondent, clarify and queries and generally help them overcome difficulties. However, it is still practical to limit the time involved with approximately 20 mins being a realistic maximum time. If much longer than this, the respondent may lose his/her concentration and/or become bored. Note, a poorly designed questionnaire can take twice as long to administer and complete as a well designed one.

Tips for Questionnaire Design

1. Write clear instructions for respondents showing by the use of an example how to complete the questionnaire. Failure to do this increases respondent error.

2. Where the questionnaire is to be administered by an interviewer the usual convention is to write the instructions for

the interviewer in CAPITAL LETTERS with the questions printed in lower case.

3. Leave a space between each question. Do not be tempted to condense the questionnaire into too few pages.

4. Leave plenty of space for written answers, particularly with open-ended questions (2-3 lines is not sufficient).

5. Try to keep different topics separate from each other. It may be useful to physically indicate a change of topic by drawing a line across the questionnaire. The respondent is then prepared for the change in content and does not become confused. Also he/she will not then try to 'match' the answer to the previous questions.

6. If the topics covered appear totally unconnected a short sentence introducing each one is reassuring for respondents.

7. Try to make subject changes as logical as possible so that the questionnaire appears to 'flow' and does not appear to 'jump backwards and forwards'

8. Marking each section with a symbol such as *, X, can make data analysis quicker, particularly if you have help with the analysis from someone not as familiar as you are with the project.

9. If you decide to use coloured paper make sure it is not too dark a colour as this can make reading the questions difficult. Some researchers use different colours for different sections to facilitate identification for analysis.

Order and Wording of Questions

At this point you need to begin to think about how you are going to analyse the data you collect, which questions can provide raw figures that can be used to give overall views and which need to be more detailed. The questions will need to be designed to provide the type of information that you require in a form that is easily accessible.

Research appreciation

1. Keep the questions simple. Questions that are complicated and difficult to answer tend to discourage respondents. If you find that you have written a complex question because of the data that you need, try to break it down into two or three simple ones.

2. Start with easy questions such as basic background details. These are easy to complete and provide positive encouragements for respondents.

3. Questions should initially be general with the more specific issues being discussed further down the questionnaire.

4. Avoid referring back to previous questions particularly if they are not on the same page

5. Remember that the order of questions may influence the answers that you get. A simple rule is to ask behaviour patterns before attitudes as once an attitude is given the respondent may feel the need to alter their behaviour to suit their expressed attitude.

6. Be aware that if you have several questions together that need 'yes' 'no' answers some people will naturally tick the same answer to all the questions. If the issues seem similar, answers can become automatic rather than thought through. Try to minimise this by varying the wording.

7. Filter questions may save a considerable amount of your time. These are usually questions that initially start with a general yes/no and depending on the answer the respondent is 'filtered' onto the next part of the questionnaire. For example:

    Do you have any children   yes ☐ please answer
                                      questions 2, 3, and 4
                                no ☐ please go to question 5

8. When deciding on the actual words to use remember that questions need to be clear, precise and unambiguous. Meanings should be straightforward and should not be difficult to understand. For example:

    For '*acquaint*' use '*tell*' or '*inform*'

What can you find out?

For '*assist*' use '*help*'

For '*consider*' use '*think*' etc.

9. There are many standard questions covering income, occupation, age, marital status, education, type of housing, family size etc. that you will see on questionnaire after questionnaire because the information that is needed is fairly standard and you may find it easier to use some of these rather than spend time designing virtually identical questions.

Things to Avoid When Designing Questions

1. Ambiguous questions. Only refer to one thing at a time. Avoid words that can have two meanings. For example does 'you' mean the singular or the plural, does 'country' mean 'countryside' or 'nationality'?

2. Can the meaning be altered if emphasis is place in a different part of the sentence. For example 'why do you say that?' can be read in different ways.

3. Questions that are too long. The respondent may have forgotten the beginning by the time they have reached the end, and this means that your answer may be based only on the last half of the question.

4. Don't ask questions that really need two answers. For example:

   Do you know what the local authority's policy regarding education is, and if so do you think that it should be changed?

5. Leading questions which presuppose the answer. For example:

   You are not in favour of the law changing are you?

6. Loaded questions which bias the respondents answer because they indicate what is the 'normal' response. For example:

   Most people support the bill against experiments on human embryos. What are your views?

7. Avoid using negative or double negatives as these questions need much more thinking about. For example:

The law on abortion should not be changed
☐ yes
☐ no

8. Do not ask apologetic questions. If you feel the need to apologise about the question the respondent will pick up your attitude and may resent or refuse to answer the question. Be matter of fact and either ask the question or leave it out.

9. Don't ask questions that require memory feats as you cannot assume that the respondents' memory will be accurate.

10. If you need to ask questions on sensitive or embarrassing subjects make the question as objective as you can, and ask these questions towards the end of the questionnaire because if they upset the respondent and he/she decides not to answer any more questions you will have lost minimal data. Asked at the beginning it may mean that you end up with several questionnaires which only have one to two questions answered.

11. Avoid 'jargon' and emotive terms like 'scrounger' and 'trouble maker', and terms that have a status value like 'residence' instead of 'house'

All you have to do now is put together a package which includes, the letter explaining the project, the questionnaire and a stamped addressed envelope. These can then be mailed to the chosen sample.

Interviewing

This method has several advantages when compared to questionnaire administration. For instance, you can note facial expression, gestures, hesitation etc. Also you can explore issues raised and discuss attitudes, feelings and beliefs more easily. However you must remember that interviews are time consuming and therefore this method of data collection is only suitable for relatively small groups. You may have decided that for your project interviews would be more likely to provide the information that you need, but to make sure that you do not just end up chatting to your respondent. You need to decide exactly what type of interview you wish to conduct and then design a suitable interview schedule.

Basically there are three kinds of interview:

1. structured
2. semi-structured
3. unstructured

1. Structured interviews

A structured interview is one where all the questions are predetermined but respondents are asked each question by an interviewer. Although this method does allow expression and hesitation etc to be registered together with the inclusion of some comments, the rigidity of the interview schedule is such that the interviewer has little freedom to pursue ideas or issues that arise during the interview. However, if you want to collect mainly factual information but believe interviews (perhaps because of literacy, or language barriers) would be more effective than a questionnaire, then this is probably the right type of interview to use. Also if you are unused to interviewing, this is a good method to start with as the structure ensures that you are not side-tracked and that you do not miss out any vital issues.

2 Semi-Structured interviews

As the name suggests, these interviews whilst they do still have some structure which ensures that all major topics are covered, are less formal and give interviewers more freedom to gather a wider range of information. The use of broad areas that can be expanded upon means that, although some answers can be readily recorded others cannot be. You might like to consider using a tape recorder as conversation is rather inhibited if the interviewer is frantically writing down everything that is said. Inevitably, you will either lose some of the data, or by asking the respondent to slow down or repeat their answers you will break their train of though thus limiting the information gained. This is a good method to use for most projects where interviewing is chosen because of the range and depth of information that can be gathered. Also, even if you are not used to conducting interviews, you will still be able to make sure that the information you gather is relevant.

If you have decided to use either structured or semi-structured interviews for your project, then the preparation for interviewing follows the same initial steps described earlier in this chapter in questionnaire design. However, there is one important difference. Once you have devised your questions and are sure that you have avoided the pitfalls of question design, you will need to look again at each question. This is because written English is different from spoken English and your questions would be stilted and unreal if used in the written format. Consequently, you now have to put each question into spoken English. Check carefully that when you do this you do not introduce bias again and make sure that you mark on each question where the emphasis of the sentence is to come. For example:

*Can you tell me **why** you think it is important*

The different meaning given by the different emphasis could cause big variations in the data you collect for example:

Why *do you say that?*

Why do **you** *say that?*

Why do you say **that***?*

As you can see the difference in emphasis means that the respondent will concentrate their answer on a different aspect of the question; hence you will not have standard data.

Remember that, with semi-structured interviewing, the questions are really prompts covering key areas and you may not need to ask them all if respondents cover the material in answers to earlier questions.

3 Unstructured Interviews

Tape recorders are essential for this type of interview as you do not have a clear schedule and this is the hardest type of interview to use unless you have considerable experience. Because it has no real format, it is also very easy for the respondent to launch off into a pet theme with the interviewer desperately trying to regain control of the session. For instance, a colleague who has considerable experience in interviewing decided to use unstructured interviewing for her latest project. She changed her mind after an exhausting first interview which lasted over three and a half hours and still did not covered all the areas she wanted to discuss.

In practice, unstructured interviews are rarely used in isolation (Burgess 1984). Instead, they are combined with another method such as observation. In these circumstances they can be extremely useful in enabling the researcher to gain information not otherwise available and may give an indication as to why a particular behaviour pattern observed by the researcher actually occurred (Burgess 1981).

If you decide to use this method, it is sensible to provide yourself with a 'visual aid' to help you gather appropriate information. This is usually a short topic list of the main issues that you wish to cover. Using this you can check that you are covering the major points for your study. Oakley (1981) suggests this type of interview is particularly useful for feminist and contentious issues, so although you have to accept that these interviews are often much longer and much more complex to analyse, you may still decide that they are the most suitable for your project.

Setting the Scene

Whichever type of interview you decide to use, setting the scene appropriately is essential, because if your respondent is not at ease, the conversation will be stilted and limited. So let's consider the essential elements of the interview setting.

1. The actual place that you use, should be quiet and if it has large windows, you need to think about two things. Firstly, the sun shining directly onto anyone can be distressing. Therefore, you need to remember what time of day you will be interviewing. Secondly, if the chairs are placed looking out of the window, it is almost inevitable that something will happen to distract your respondent (such as a lorry unloading, or a game of football) and you may get some vague and possibly inappropriate answers.

2. The chairs should be of similar type and height as you wish to create a relaxed atmosphere not one of subordinate/dominant. For the same reason, it is better not to sit behind a desk, and not to have the chairs directly opposite one another.

3. Respondents need to know approximately how long the interview will last because they need to fit the interview around their other commitments.

4. Whichever method of interviewing you choose to use, you need to plan how to record carefully. If you have decided to take notes, practice a method of shorthand that you understand (don't try to learn a professional system - it takes more time and effort than you realise). Nothing is more off putting to a respondent than an interviewer who frantically takes notes and has no time to make eye contact or to respond to the answers given. If you have decided to use a tape recorder, use one with a microphone so that the actual machine does not need to sit obtrusively between you. Do use good quality tapes or your recording will be blurred.

Observation Studies

Although all types of observation are usually described under one heading, this is not strictly correct. There are different types of observation methods that you can use to gather information, and the projects that they are used for differ considerably. For this reason the two main types, nonparticipant and participant observation, will be discussed separately.

1 Nonparticipant Observation

This type of data collection is useful when you want to study a particular social setting. The researcher is not part of the setting, instead the idea is to look at and describe the setting (Brown, 1989). For example you may want to make changes in an outpatient clinic, but you need to be sure that the changes are necessary, and that they will improve the overall service provided. You are going to use direct observation of a social setting to provide a picture of the clinic and make decisions about the future running of this clinic.

What can you find out?

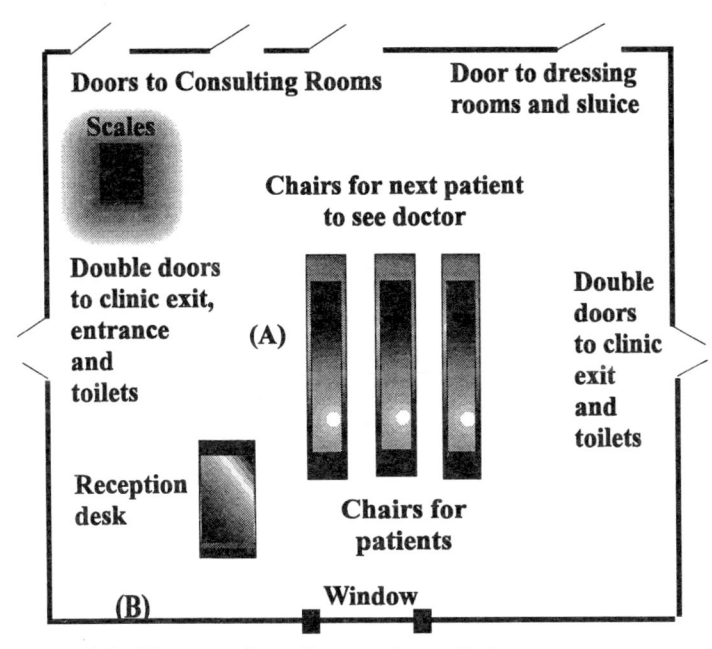

```
┌─────────────────────────────────────────────────┐
│  Doors to Consulting Rooms   Door to dressing   │
│                              rooms and sluice   │
│   Scales                                        │
│                                                 │
│                  Chairs for next patient        │
│                      to see doctor              │
│  Double doors                                   │
│  to clinic exit,                    Double      │
│  entrance      (A)                  doors       │
│  and                                to clinic   │
│  toilets                            exit        │
│                                     and         │
│                                     toilets     │
│                                                 │
│  Reception                                      │
│  desk                                           │
│                    Chairs for                   │
│                     patients                    │
│                      Window                     │
│   (B)                                           │
└─────────────────────────────────────────────────┘
```

Figure 6.2: Observation: Out-patient clinic

For this to be an effective exercise you need to find some way to observe and note down everything that happens without your presence affecting the way the people in the clinic behave. As Bell (1987) points out his is not any easy option, but carried out carefully it has the advantage of showing you exactly what happens, not what staff and patients say happens. You will need to find somewhere that enables you to see all of the clinic but is not obtrusive. Look at Figure 6.2. Would you sit in space (A) or (B)?

75

Research appreciation

If the researcher sits in spot (A) he or she will be immediately apparent to everyone entering the clinic and this may well affect the behaviour patterns observed. If however he or she sits in place (B), the major areas of the clinic can be seen but the researcher appears to be part of the overall setting and can unobtrusively watch and record the whole clinic. You have to accept that if your are doing this on your own it may be difficult for you to see and record everything that happens. You need to devise a way of recording information that is quick, clear and facilitates the recording of the actions/interactions that you consider essential. So, where do you start? First brainstorm, just as you did when looking at defining the problem (see Figure 6.3). This shouldn't take you more than 10–15 mins.

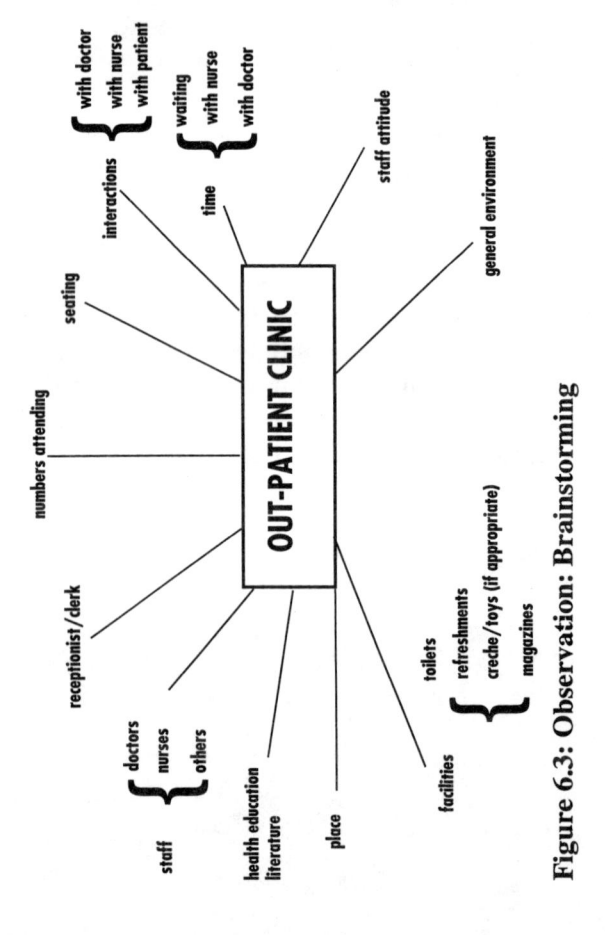

Figure 6.3: Observation: Brainstorming

What can you find out?

Next, look carefully at everything you have written and write a list with the most important factors at the top. Once this is complete start at the bottom of the list and cross off everything that is not essential. This list will form the basis of your observational data. Look at each factor and decide how you could record it. Figure 6.4 gives an example of how you could record interactions.

nurse speaks to other nurse	A1
nurse speaks to patient	A2
nurse speaks to relative	A3
nurse speaks to doctor	A4
nurse speaks to receptionist	A5
nurse answers telephone	A6
nurse listens to other nurse	B1
nurse listens to patients	B2
nurse listens to relative	B3
nurse listens to doctor	B4
nurse listens to receptionist	B5
and so on	

Figure 6.4 Example of a Way to Record Interactions

Research appreciation

When you have considered every item on the list, you have the basis of a recording system that you could use within an observational grid (this is a chart which is designed to let you record a variety of different information rapidly and easily).

It is important that before you go on to design the actual grid, you are happy with the way you have decided to record data because once you start your observation you will have no time to reconsider. If you find using numbers confusing choose symbols or letters, but make sure that you can learn the categories easily as you will have to remember them all.

Designing a grid that is easy to use is vital as otherwise your data will be sketchy and inaccurate. At this point you may wish to look at some previously published work (Monette *et al*, 1986; Shaw, 1978; Brown, 1989). All of these show ways to record social settings. The main thing to remember is to keep it as simple as possible. To provide yourself with a grid (chart) that takes very little time to complete and which you can analyse **easily** once you have completed the field work.

Once you have decided what and how you will record your data, you have only to decide how to record the length and frequency of each action/interaction. This is the final factor which needs to go on your chart and which then completes the grid. It is usually done by dividing the time for observation into 'time-slots' often of as short a period as 3-5 seconds. Only you can decide how detailed you want to be. Suppose, for example, that your time in the clinic had shown you that there were several key areas in the clinic. You may decide to record the interactions that occur at these places. Figure 6.5 shows a grid with five second time-slots.

Place	Time				
	0–5	6–10	11–15	16–20	21–25
Reception desk					
Weighing scales					
Waiting chairs (give chair and patient a number					
Door from consulting room					
Door out of the clinic					

Figure 6.5: Observations: recording interactions in selected places

Once you have your data collection tool, you should pilot it to check that it is practical and that you have not designed something where you are too busy remembering the categories to see what is happening. If you have never used a grid before, start with one that allows you to measure one part of the setting. Only when you find it easy should you move on to try to record a wider set of variables. There is nothing more dispiriting than sitting there knowing that you are missing most of what is happening.

You must also remember that familiarity with the scene being observed may mean that you do not notice everything that happens because some actions are so familiar that you overlook them unless you are concentrating hard.

Concentration can be a major problem in observational studies. The effort of recording everything is very tiring and you should settle for repeated short periods rather than one long one. Your concentration will also be affected if you are tired, hungry, thirsty, too hot or too cold, so as far as possible, you should make sure you are 'comfortable' before you start.

When you finish each short session of observation, write notes about the session as a whole. Describe the overall time you were observing, note any types of activities not in your grid and try to present a verbal picture of the setting. Also, comment on anything that distracted you and may, therefore, have influenced your recording.

Research appreciation

2 Participant observation

Although you will still be observing what is happening, this method is very different to that described above, because for this type of observation you need to join in. You are no longer the observer looking on but a participating member of the group being observed. Unlike direct observation, you cannot just decide which settings need observing and start. For this method you can either be part of the group before you start your project, ie. you may wish to study the nursing care provided on the ward you work in, or you can join a group, (eg. the staff on the ward you want to study) wait until you have been fully accepted and then try to analyse what is happening. Also, for the group to act naturally, in participant observation the group being studies is not usually aware of the researchers role. They see you only as a member of the group. Both these options mean that projects take some time to carry out and there is always the risk that the researcher will become so involved in the group that he or she will be unable to see any viewpoint other than that of the group. Hence, their findings will be biased.

It is very difficult to maintain objective recordings when fully immersed in the setting and, unlike non-participant observation, you do not have the luxury of recording as things happen. Notes have to be written when possible in the most concise and unobtrusive way and transcribed (re-written) as soon as possible afterwards (Burgess, 1981). We call such notes 'field notes'. Brainstorming and devising a simple grid can help but the time-slots will have to be different. Certainly, you could not hope to record every five seconds and remain a participating member of a group. However, you should accept that your notes should be transcribed into longhand at the end of each period with the group. If you do not do this, then the following sessions with the group may influence your notes and you will transcribe what you **think** happened rather than what actually happened. As with non-participant observation, you should also write notes about the session as a whole to support your observations.

Whichever method of observation you choose to use, for nurses there is another aspect which cannot be ignored. What do you do if you see unsafe practice? For example, what would you do if you saw an intravenous drip running through? Your Code of Conduct and your professionalism mean that you cannot just ignore such incidents and you should decide before starting the project where the boundaries of acceptable practice lie, what you think you would find acceptable, and at which point you would find it necessary to intervene. You should then discuss this with your manager or the manager of the area/setting you wish to study and gain their agreement for your decession. Remember, once you have intervened, you may have permanently altered what happens, or in the case of participant observation terminated the project, as your true role of researcher will have been highlighted and it would be difficult for the group to accept you as a 'normal member'.

References

Bell J (1987). *Doing Your research Project*, Open University Press, Milton Keynes

Brown R (1989). *Individualised Care: **The Role of The Ward Sister***, RCN Research series:Scutari Press, Harrow

Burgess R G (1981). Keeping a research diary, *Camb J Educ*, **11**:1, 75-83

Burgess R G (1984). *In The Field*, Unwin Hyman, London.

Hoinville G, Jowell, R et al (1978). *Survey Research Practice*, Heinemann, London

Moser C A, Kalton G (1978). *Survey Methods in Social Investigation*, Heinemann, London.

Oakley A (1981). Interviewing Women. In Roberts H. (ed), *A Contradiction in Terms*, Routledge and Keegan Paul, London.

Oppenheim A N (1990). *Questionnaire Design and Attitude Measurement*, Heinemann, London.

Phillips D R (1981). *Do-It-Yourself Social Surveys*, The Polytechnic of North London.

Chapter 7
What Can You Do With It?

You have reached the point of wanting to analyse and present your finding and chapters seven, eight and nine have been designed to help you do this. By the end of these next chapters you should be able to:

1   decide which type of analysis best suits your findings
2   carry out basic analysis and present your findings both graphically and descriptively
3   write a report on your project

Throughout this book we have talked about 'data', but what do we mean by the term data.
Data is information and it includes:
- completed questionnaires
- fields notes/reports
- recorded interviews
- video recordings
- official/national records/surveys

All of the above can be collected using research methods, but without careful study they cannot easily be used to contribute to knowledge and understanding. This process is analysis.

There are different methods of analysing data but these divide broadly into two categories - **quantitative** and **qualitative**. Quantitative data analysis is concerned with numerical measurement and will be the basis for this chapter. Analysing qualitative data will be discussed in chapter 8.

Research appreciation

This type of analysis can be used in two ways:

a) to describe

This is the summarising of data (information) so that it is more usable. The researcher is able to see if relationships (patterns/links) exist between variables. However some information is inevitably lost by this method and it is possible to obtain results that can be misleading.

b) to infer

This involves either making generalisations about a particular population on the basis of a sample drawn from that population, or formulating general laws on the basis of repeated observations.

Levels of measurement

Most social researchers refer to the way we categorise the data they have collected as measurement. It is usual for different categories measurements to be given numerical labels, and this can result in findings with several different types of properties. These findings or 'scales' are referred to as different levels of measurement. We use four main scales:

Nominal

This is the simplest scale and is used when all that can be said about these numbered categories is that they are mutually exclusive and exhaustive (ie. one individual can only belong to one category).

Example of a nominal scale

Question asked = What is your religion?

The researcher would use a set of categories, such as the following to record the replies.

1	Catholic	2.	Protestant	3	Christian other
4	Jewish	5	Muslim	6	Other
7	None	8	Unclassifiable	9	No answer

Note that number 8 means that the researcher did not understand the respondent's reply, or it was too ambiguous to fit into any of the other categories. In analysis number 8 and 9 therefore tend to be classified as missing data and are not frequently used. Consideration of numbers 1–7 show that the order used was arbitrary and that the numeric labels can only be used for simple procedures such as counting how many belong to each category, finding percentages, identifying the most commonly occurring group etc.

Ordinal

With this level of measurement, as the name suggests, the numbers can be used to put results in rank order.

Example of an ordinal scale
In athletics at the end of a race the competitors could be ranked as follows

1.	David
2.	John
3.	Michael
4.	Ian

This shows that David beat John but not by how much he beat John. It is possible to say that if David beat Michael and Michael beat Ian, David also beat Ian. In general however, the usual arithmetical processes of addition, subtraction, multiplication and division cannot be used and so, again, the information gained by analysis is limited.

Interval

The third type of data is referred to as interval data. Again, the name gives an idea of the characteristics of the data. With an interval scale the relationship between the assigned numbers and the observed categories is such that the differences between the given numbers are constant and have meaning, even though the scale values themselves are arbitrary.

Example of an interval scale
   The Fahrenheit Scale for measuring temperature.

Ratio
If it is possible to locate an absolute or non-arbitrary zero on the scale, the level of measurement is said to be a ratio scale and the ratios are meaningful as well as the differences between the points (the intervals).

Example of a ratio scale
   A birth rate is a ratio scale because birth rate of 40 per 1,000 is twice one of 20 per 1,000.

With the last two types of data, far more calculations are possible, and traditionally we start with what are usually called '**measures of central tendency**'. You will have come across at least one of these although you probably didn't use this name because we usually talk about '**averages**'.

The term 'average' is usually used to mean a typical value. However, this common usage means that it is used in a wide variety of different contexts and therefore the meaning of this term is neither standard nor precise. Averages are used in the analysis of data but in very specific ways. In research, we are much more precise about using terms and we always refer to measures of central tendency not averages.

Three terms of central tendency are used:-

   Mean, Median, Mode.

Mean This is the version of central tendency with which you will probably be most familiar as you will have come across it when you did arthmetic at school. It is calculated by adding up all the individual numbers and dividing by the total number in the sample.

Median Usually this is said to be the mid point of frequencies of observations or categories found when they have been arranged according to rank or size, so 50% of values lay above and 50% lay below.

What can you do with your data?

Mode This is simply the most frequently occurring observation(s)

Let's consider how you could calculate each of these. Supposing you wanted to look at the results of a screening programme for children with a particular disorder. The screening programme started in 1981 and you want to study the years 1981–87

These are the numbers of children screened:-

Year	1981	1982	1983	1984	1985	1986	1987
Children Screened	10	7	8	7	9	10	2

The easiest of the three measures to calculate is the **mode**. Remember this is the most frequently occurring figure. In our example, the most frequent occurring number is 10, so,

the mode is 10

The second measure to consider is the median. Remember, the median is the mid point, so 50% of the findings lay below the median and 50% lay above, and it is **not** simply the middle point in the range. So, in our example:
First list the observations in rank order

Year	1987	1982	1984	1983	1985	1981	1986
Children Screened	2	3	7	8	9	10	10

Next, we need to find the year that is the midpoint. If you look at the list in rank order, you will see that the year where 50% of the groups lie below and 50% lie above is 1983.

the median is 8

The mean is calculated by:

using the list of all children screened as above

adding together all the observations (ie. how many were screened altogether)

For our example:

$$10 + 3 + 8 + 7 + 9 + 10 + 2 = 49$$

dividing the number of observations by the number of occasions (ie. in this case 7 different occasions)

$$\frac{49}{7} = 7$$

Therefore, for this example **the mean is 7**

You will now be able to work out each of these measures. It is often easier to use them if they are presented graphically as below:-

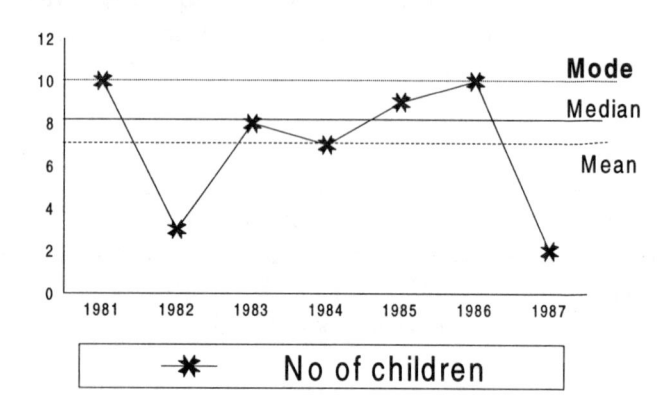

[Graph showing No of children across years 1981-1987 with values approximately 10, 3, 8, 7, 9, 10, 2, with horizontal lines indicating Mode (10), Median (8), and Mean (7)]

Figure 7.1: Mode, Median and Mean

As you can see this clearly shows the differences between all measures. Always check that you know which one you want to use.

The mode is perhaps more useful when there are a large number of cases and the data has been grouped.

Using Charts and Graphs to Present Data

So far we have described the types of data and outlined how you can start to analyse it, as our last example showed an equally important question is how to present it. You may want to illustrate your finding with charts or graphs. One of the simplest ways of presenting data is to use a pie chart. This is a circular representation of the facts and is not suitable for all types of information as it gives a pictorial comparison of each component part of the total picture at one point in time only.

It is most useful for figures that are intended only as comparisons and do not need other calculation, for instance if your survey had looked at the number of women in your area that use each method of contraception. Suppose in that your survey you contacted 120,000 women and your sample shows the following findings.

Table 7.1: Number of Women Using Each Method of Contraception

i)	oral contraception	=	30,000	women
ii)	intra-uterine devices	=	16,800	women
iii)	diaphragms	=	10,800	women
iv)	sheath	=	30,000	women
v)	natural methods	=	12,000	women
vi)	pregnant or trying to become pregnant	=	20,400	women
	Total	=	120,000	women

For this type of result a pie chart would be very effective, so where do you start? There are several distinct stages that you need to go through to produce your chart

1. List all the categories that make up the whole sample: in this case:
    - i) oral contraception
    - ii) intra-uterine devices
    - iii) diaphragms
    - iv) sheath
    - v) natural methods
    - vi) pregnant or trying to become pregnant

Research appreciation

2) Add all these categories together to find the total number of women in the sample

In this example we know the number of women in each category (See Table 7.1)

3) Now express each category as a percentage of the whole sample.

Remember percentages are worked out using the following equations:

$$\frac{individual\ category}{total\ number} \times 100$$

So for this example:

i) oral contraception = $\frac{30000}{120000} \times 100 = 25$

ii) intra-uterine device = $\frac{16800}{120000} \times 100 = 14$

iii) diaphragm = $\frac{10800}{120000} \times 100 = 9$

iv) sheath = $\frac{30000}{120000} \times 100 = 25$

v) natural methods = $\frac{12000}{120000} \times 100 = 10$

vi) pregnant or trying to become pregnant = $\frac{20400}{120000} \times 100 = 17$

Total = 100

4). The data is now ready to be presented in the form of a pie chart, and for this you will need a protractor and a compass.

5) Look carefully at the protractor, you will see that it is marked into degrees and that there are 360 degrees in a circle. So to work out the size of each portion of the pie chart you need to know one more equation, again based round percentages. This equation tells you how many of the total 360 degrees each of your groups will use.

The total percentage = 100
The total number of degrees = 360
so each 1% = 360 : = 3.60 degrees

Therefore, the degrees for each category are:

i)	oral contraception	=	3.6	x	25	=	90
ii)	intra-uterine device	=	3.6	x	14	=	50.4
iii)	diaphragm	=	3.6	x	9	=	32.4
iv)	sheath	=	3.6	x	25	=	90
v)	natural methods	=	3.6	x	10	=	36
vi)	pregnant or trying to become pregnant	=	3.6	x	17	=	61.2

6) Now using the compass draw a circle and mark the centre with a dot. Using this draw a diameter and using this as a base line plot your chart using the protractor. Figure 7.2 shows the completed pie chart.

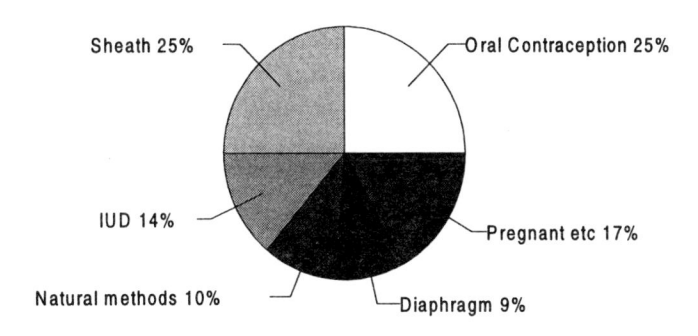

Figure 7.2: Pie chart showing contraception usage

Although pie charts are very useful for comparing individual categories to the sample as a whole, if you look back at the pie chart

Research appreciation

you can see that although the sections are of different size, because only the chart and not the original figures are included you have to guess the actual differences, accuracy is not really possible. So if you want to go on to compare the various categories with each other, a simple table or a bar chart is usually regarded as more effective.

If we decide to look at the same example and present the finding using a table we go back to the original list of figures:

Number of Women Using Each method of Contraception

- i) oral contraception
- ii) intra-uterine devices
- iii) diaphragms
- iv) sheath
- v) natural methods
- vi) pregnant or trying to become pregnant

Table 7.2: Express these figures as a table of numbers

Type of Contraception	No of Women	% of Sample
oral contraception	30,000	25
intra-uterine devices	16,800	14
diaphragm	10,800	9
sheath	30,000	25
natural methods	12,000	10
pregnant or trying for pregnancy	20,400	17
Total	120,000	100

This type of presentation still does not actually show the difference in size between the different categories; you have to carefully study the figures and mentally calculate the differences. A bar chart has the advantage that the differences can be seen immediately. The figures can be plotted on a bar chart, either in their original format or in percentages

What can you do with your data?

The chart is plotted by first drawing the x and y axis as for a traditional graph.

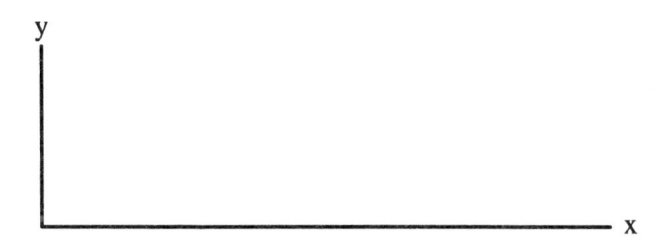

Figure 7.3: XY Axis

Using the figures in your table you can now draw two bar charts. In the first the actual figures are used and in the second the percentages.

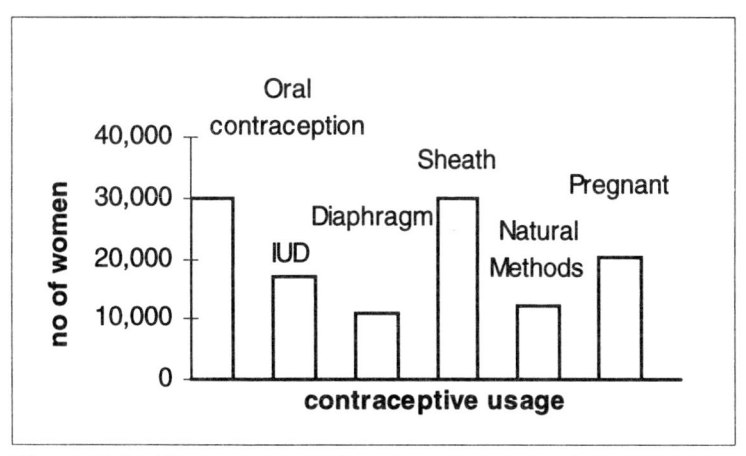

Figure 7.4a: Data presentation: bar chart showing contraceptive usage in actual numbers

Research appreciation

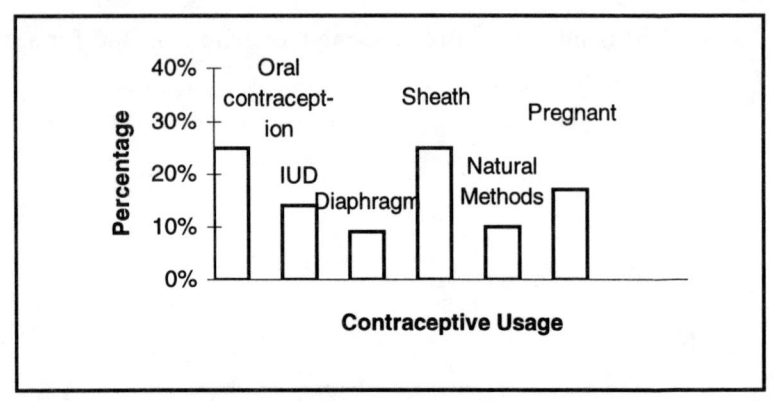

Figure 7.4b: Data presentation: bar chart showing contraceptive usage in percentage of total usage

Finally, let's look at one more kind of graph, supposing your survey included findings that had been taken over a number of years. For each method of contraception you had several figures tables. The bar chart overleaf is cumbersome. You would have to draw a separate chart for each method, use computer software to draw a multi-dimensional diagram or draw a stacked chart. So, you may decide to use a table (7.3) or to use line graphs to try to show, visually, the changing patterns over the five years. Figure 7.5 shows what this would look like.

What can you do with your data?

Table 7.3: Data presentation: table showing contraceptive usage 1985-89

Method of Contraception	No. of women in each year in thousands				
	1985	1986	1987	1988	1989
oral contraception	30	26.5	29	32	25
intra-uterine devices	16.8	18	17.5	15.8	14
diaphragm	10.8	11	11	12	125
sheath	30	28	32.6	34.6	36.2
natural methods	12	11.8	10.7	7.6	15.3
pregnant or trying for pregnancy	20.4	25.2	19.2	18	17
Total	120,000 each year				

Figure 7.5: Line & Marker Graph

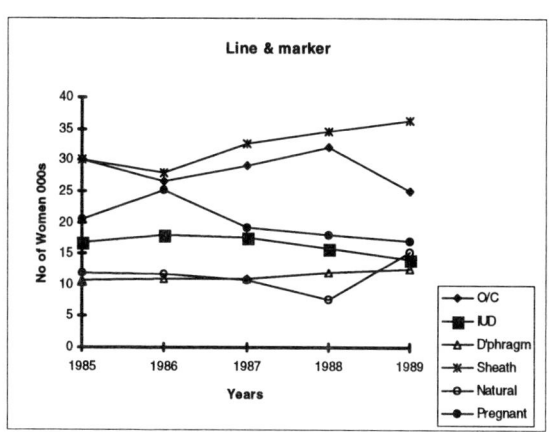

However, as you can see, this graph looks rather confused and is difficult to use if you want to compare individual methods, e.g. diaphragm and sheath, or to compare interuterine devices with oral contraception. There are several possible permutations and a series of graphs may well be more effective than one that is too complicated. All that you need to do is ensure that when you look at the graph the information that you are trying to convey is **immediately** apparent.

95

Research appreciation

at the graph the information that you are trying to convey is **immediately** apparent.

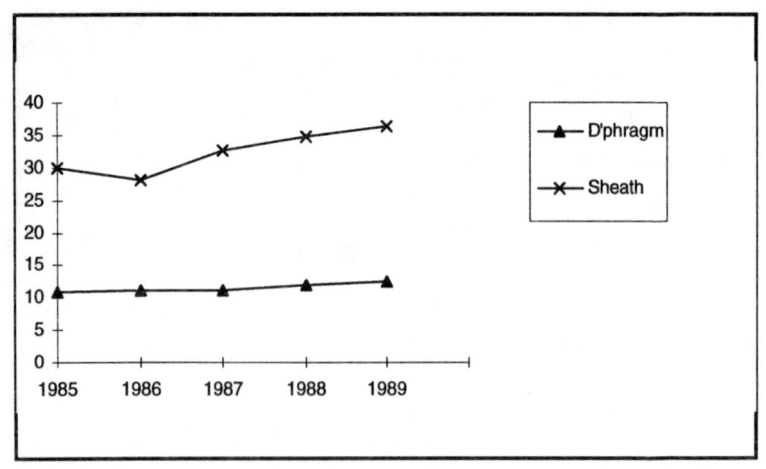

Figure 7.5a: Line and Marker Graph - Diaphragm & Sheath

You need to have more than one set of figures in a line graph and make sure that you have clearly labelled each one as shown in Figure 7.5. After all you may not be present to explain the results and your whole survey could be misinterpreted if no-one is sure which line is which.

Dispersion

Now that we've looked at some simple ways to present data we need to go on to look at some more detailed calculations that you can carry out with this kind of data. Measures of central tendency and pie charts and graphs show above whilst useful do not actually tell us a great deal about the data and we often need to know more about each set of figures (sometimes called scores/cases).

For example, if we take the mean and compare two sets of scores (Table 7.4), we can see that although they both have the same mean, they have very little else in common. In order to make a useful statement or indication from these figures, we need to find out more information.

What can you do with your data?

Table 7.4: Calculating mean scores

1)	7	3	6	9	5	mean =	6
2)	2	5	6	6	11	mean =	6

Three easy calculations which can give more insight into the characteristics of the scores are those giving:

> *range*
>
> *mean deviation*
>
> *standard deviation*

Range

This is the distance between the bottom and top scores. For Figure 1 the range is 3–9 inclusive of both scores and for Figure 2 the range is 2–11 inclusive of both scores, clearly showing differences between the two sets of figures. However, this still does not tell us how or where the individual scores are placed within the overall example, so we need to look further and consider the mean and standard deviations.

Mean and Standard Deviations

These are the terms used to describe by how much each of the values differs on average from the arithmetical mean. In other words you find out how far above or below the mean each average figure is. To do this, you follow exactly the same process as you used to find the mean. You find each individual difference and then add up these differences and divide by the number of values in your sample. Lets see how this works in practice. Use all of the scores (observations) and take the deviation (difference) of each score from the mean and then work out some kind of average of these deviations.

Look back at the example given in table 7.4 and use the first set of figures.

Research appreciation

Example of Using Table 7.4

1   List all individual scores

        7
        3
        6
        9
        5

The mean = 6

2   Calculate how much each score deviates from the mean

    7   deviates from 6 by 1, and is greater than 6 so the difference = + 1

    3   deviates from 6 by 3, and is smaller than 6 so the difference = - 3

    6   is the mean so the deviance is said to be 0

    9   deviates from 6 by 3, and is greater than 6, so the difference = + 3

    5   deviates from 6 by 1, and is smaller than 6, so the difference = - 1

We therefore have +1 -3 +0 +-1
        which = 1-3+0+3-1=0

You can see that the answer is zero because we have added up **all** differences from either side of the mean, so we have to find a way to get rid of the minuses that cancel out our answer. There are two simple ways to do this.

1   ignore the signs and take the absolute value of the differences

2   square the differences as two negatives squared automatically become positive

What can you do with your data?

Mean Deviation

The first method gives us a result that we refer to as the **mean deviation** and this can be written using an accepted formula as follows:

$$\text{mean deviation} = \frac{\text{the sum of the DIFFERENCE between each score and the arithmetic mean}}{\text{the number of scores}}$$

However, this is rather lengthy, so we convert its words to symbols: using symbols the equation looks like this:

$$\text{mean deviation} = \frac{\sum (x_i - \bar{x})}{N}$$

where S = the sum of
xi = the individual score/case
x = mean
N = number of scores/cases

Let's try using this with the first set of numbers in Table 7.4
List the scores/cases

7
3
6
9
5

Calculate how much each deviates from the mean it $(x_i - \bar{x})$ for each score/case

$7 (x_i - \bar{x}) = 7 - 6 = 1$
$3 (x_i - \bar{x}) = 3 - 6 = -3$
$6 (x_i - \bar{x}) = 6 - 6 = 0$
$9 (x_i - \bar{x}) = 9 - 6 = 3$
$5 (x_i - \bar{x}) = 5 - 6 = -1$

but we are ignoring the minus signs so our sum is

$1 + 3 + 0 + 3 + 1 = 8$

$$\text{mean deviation} = \frac{8}{N}$$

N = 5 as there are 5 scores/cases so the mean deviation

$$= \frac{8}{5} = 1.6$$

99

Research appreciation

To make sure you understand this work out the mean deviation for the second example in table 7.4 (2), page 97.

The mean deviation = (*answer at end of chapter, page 117*)

Unfortunately the mean deviation has serious disadvantages:

1. absolute values are not easily manipulated algebraically
2. it is not easily interpreted theoretically – this is the most serious disadvantage.
3. it does not lead to simple mathematical results.

So, although mean deviation may be adequate for simple descriptive purposes as it gives you an indication of the **average** difference between individual scores or cases, it is rarely used in social science research because of the above disadvantages. Instead, we use the second method which gives us the Standard Deviation.

Standard Deviation

This uses the second method described on page 97. To arrive at a final result we have chosen to cancel out the negative signs by **squaring** all the figures and we will consequently have a much larger answer than we want. So, to cancel the effect, we reverse the calculation. Where we had multiplied each number by itself (squaring) so we now divide the number we have calculated by itself (the square root). Thus our equation this time is:

standard deviation = *the square root of*: $\dfrac{\text{the sum of the difference between individual scores and the mean squared}}{\text{the total number of scores}}$

Again, this is too long, so we convert it to symbols and the equation looks like this:

$$\text{Standard deviation} = \sqrt{\dfrac{\sum (x_1 - \bar{x})^2}{N}}$$

Where Σ = the sum of
x_1 = the individual score/case
$\bar{x}$ = the mean
N = the number of scores/cases
$\sqrt{}$ = the square root

What can you do with your data?

Note: $(x_1 - \bar{x})$ is sometimes written as d
In that case:

$$\text{Standard deviation} = \sqrt{\frac{d^2}{N}}$$

Let us look at the first example from figure 7.4 again and this time work out the standard deviation

List all the scores

7
3
6
9
5

Calculate the deviance from the mean for each score

for 7 $(x_1 - \bar{x}) = 1$
for 3 $(x_1 - \bar{x}) = -3$
for 6 $(x_1 - \bar{x}) = 0$
for 9 $(x_1 - \bar{x}) = 3$
for 5 $(x_1 - \bar{x}) = -1$

Now square each individual deviation

1 = 1
-3 = 9
0 = 0
3 = 9
-1 = 1

Add all these figures together

1 + 9 + 0 + 9 + 1 = 20

Divide by N, the number of scores/cases. In this example there are 5.

$$\text{Standard deviation} = \sqrt{\frac{20}{5}} = \sqrt{4} = 2$$

To make sure you understand this, work out the standard deviation for the second example in figure 7.4, (2) page 97.

Standard deviation = (*answers are at the end of the chapter, page 117*)

101

Research appreciation

Usually the standard deviation is written as SD for statistical examples and $\sum$ when referring to a sample population. You may also see the formula written as

$$= \sqrt{\frac{\sum (x_i - \bar{x})^2}{(N-1)}}$$

Using (N - 1) instead of (N) is because in sampling terms it is generally accepted that this reduces the bias when considering a population sample, particularly if the sample is small.

Note the formula without the square root sign eg:

$$= \frac{(x_i - \bar{x})^2}{N}$$

may be referred to as the **variance**. Mathematicians find this concept to be useful theoretically and you will often see it used in research reports.

What else you do with the standard deviation?

One of the most important uses of the standard deviation is linked to the distribution of observations around a central point. We know that most samples drawn from the population as a whole tend to follow a similar pattern so we refer to this as the "Normal Curve of Distribution" (sometimes called the Gaussian Curve). Figure 7.5 shows a normal curve of distribution.

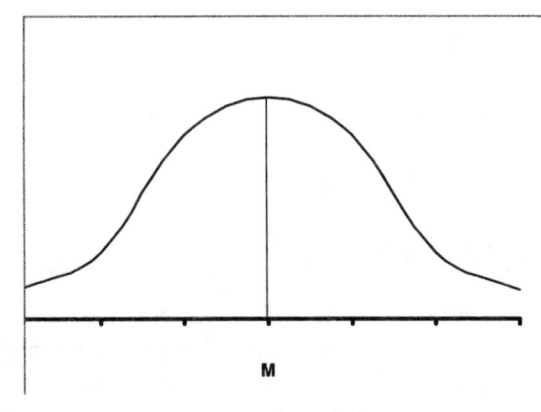

Figure 7.5: Normal curve of distribution

What can you do with your data?

If you think back to the bar chart you can see that a normal curve of distribution can be shown as a bar chart with the central point of each column joined to make a single line - much as you draw a line graph.

We know that if the results can be plotted so that they form a normal curve of distribution we can use the standard deviation in the following way:

1. Draw the normal curve of distribution
2. Mark the mean on the curve
3. Next look at the standard deviation and work out where on the bottom axis this would be if you start at the mean and go both ways. We call this one standard deviation
   68% of the population lies within this area
4. Repeat the process and we now have two marks either side of the mean. We call this two standard deviations; 95% of the population lies within this area. This is illustrated in Figure 7.6.

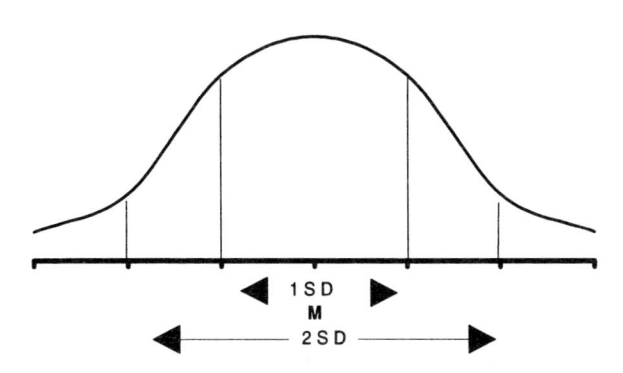

Figure 7.6: Standard Deviation

This means that provided your sample follows a normal curve of distribution, you can look in detail at different groups within your sample. You can pick out 68% or 95% if you want, i.e. look at majority findings. Or you can look at the respondents from the

Research appreciation

extreme ends of the graph. Figure 7.7 shows how you can divide your results into smaller percentages for study

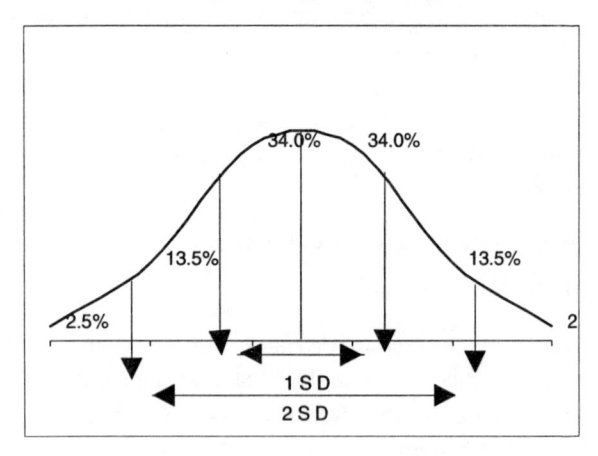

Figure 7.7: Chart showing smaller percentage studies

However, if your sample does not produce a curve like that shown in figure 7.7, but is instead 'skewed', you cannot use this approach.

What do we mean by skewed?....This is when your graph looks like either figure 7.8 or 7.9.

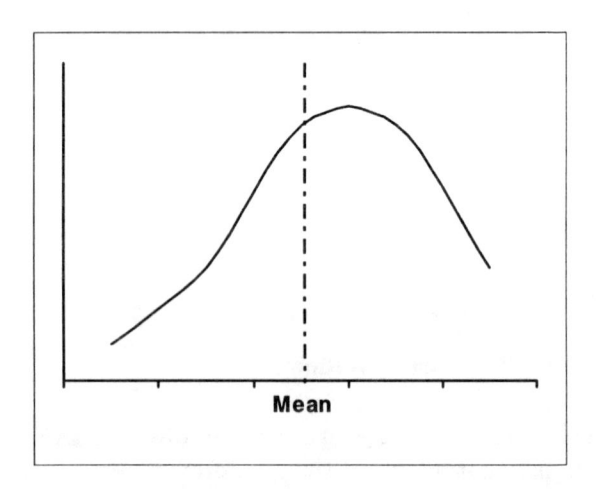

Figure 7.8: Left-hand skew (also called negative skew)

What can you do with your data?

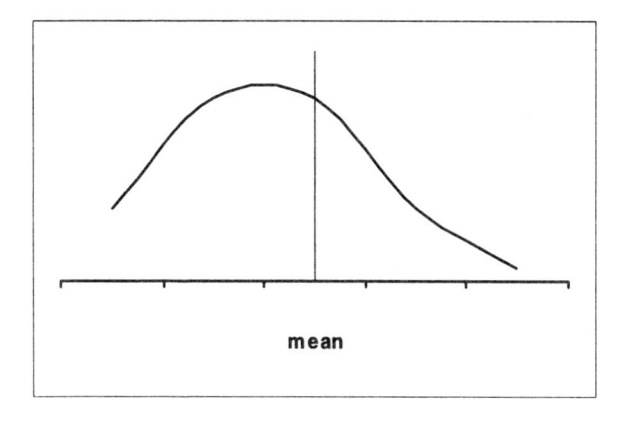

Figure 7.9: Right-hand skew (also called positive skew)

You may even find that your results do not resemble a normal curve at all and, if this is the case, you may find that to revert to a simple chart as shown in 7.10a & b is better. Always look for the most effective way to present your date, not necessarily the most complicated.

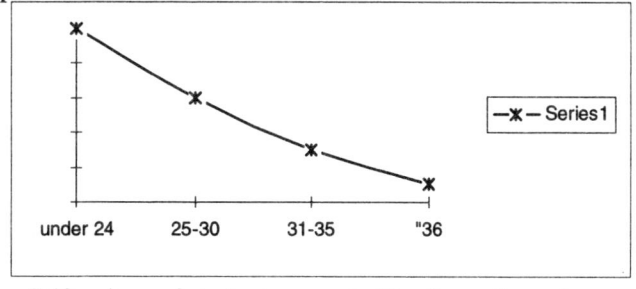

Figure 7.10a: Ages of student nurses in X college of nursing

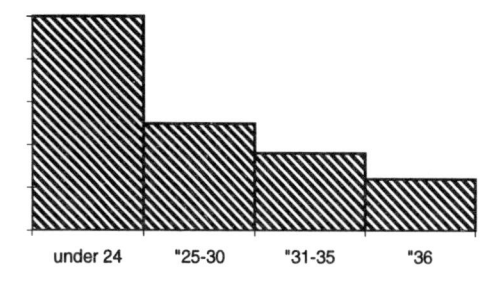

Figure 7.10b: Ages of student nurses in X college of nursing

105

Correlations

Well, what else can you do with this data? You can look for **relationships** between the variables (characteristics) in your group. For example you may have looked at height and weight, and wondered if any links are co-incidental or if they do 'co-relate'. We have already looked at plotting graphs. When you create a graph, if it looks like figure 7.11 you **appear** to have, what we call, a strong positive correlation.

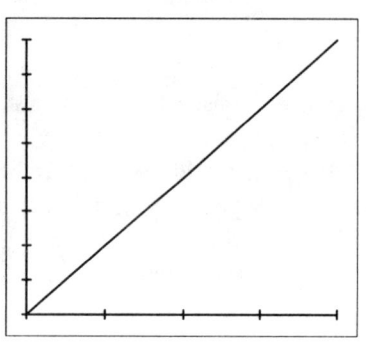

Figure 7.11: A strong positive correlation

If your graph looks like figure 7.12 you appear to have, what we call, a strong negative correlation.

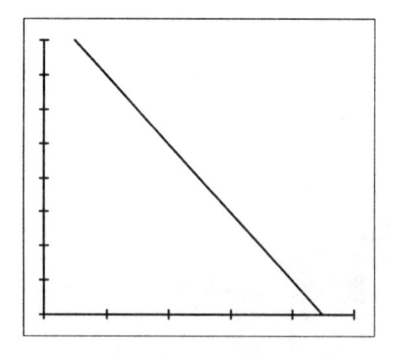

Figure 7.12: Strong negative correlation

What can you do with your data?

The terms positive and negative **only** indicate which way the graph would be. One is **not** better than the other. The perfect (straight line) positive correlation is said to be +1 and the perfect (straight line) negative correlation is said to be -1. Correlation can never be greater than ±1. However, in reality you are unlikely to get a perfectly straight line in either direction. You are more likely to get a graph, or scattergram that looks like figure 7.13 or 7.14.

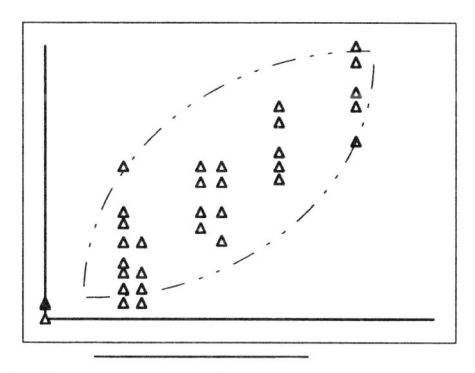

Figure 7.13: Scattergram (a)

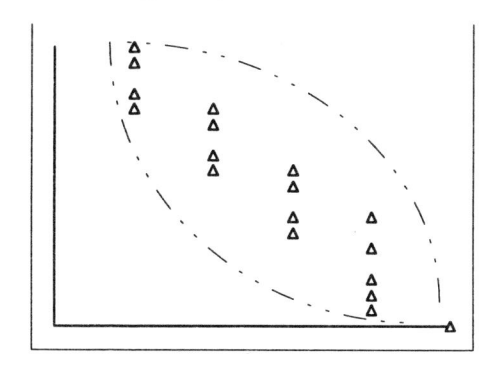

Figure 7.14: Scattergram (b)

The more scattered the data, the weaker the correlation until it looks like figure 7.15 when there is little or zero correlation.

Research appreciation

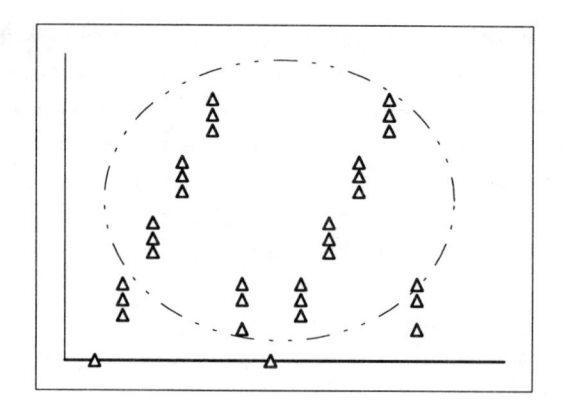

Figure 7.15: Little or zero correlation

So the nearer the correlation is to zero, the weaker the correlation

Spearman's rank order correlation

If you are working with small numbers (up to 30) one test that you can work out with the aid of a calculator is 'Spearman's rank order correlation.

Suppose you wanted to look at whether the number of times a patient attends outpatients affects their satisfaction with the service offered. First you ask each patient to record how many times they have attended and then you ask them to record on a scale of 1–5 their satisfaction with the service.

You then draw up a table that shows:

1   Patient number

2   Their satisfaction score

3   Their position in a table that ranks satisfaction scores with most satisfied as 1 and least satisfied as 6 (as there are six patients)

What can you do with your data?

Table 7.5: Patient attendance and satisfaction rating

Patient No	No of times attended clinic	Satisfaction rating	Ranked order of satisfaction
1	2	3	4
2	3	3	4
3	5	5	1
4	6		2
5	8	2	6
6	9	3	4

1 = highly dissatisfied   4 = satisfied
2 = dissatisfied   5 = highly satisfied
3 = reasonable

Note: In our examples, there is no third position. In everyday activities where more than one number is shared, we give the same value to all, but we usually give the upper score, eg. in a race where two people tie for third place we give them both third place and the next person is fifth. For this test, the rules are slightly different. In the example above rank 1 and 2 are clear, but three patients have the same score of 3 and here we average out the rank – in the same way that we find arithmetic means. The ranks that these three patients occupy are 3, 4 and 5 (the final patient is sixth in rank) so we add 3+4+5 and divide by 3 as these are three scores. Thus the average rank is:

$$\frac{3+4+5}{3} = \frac{12}{3} = 4$$

Now, like other statistical tests, Spearmans rank order correlation has a standard formula or equation and, as with the formula for standard deviation, you do not need to know how this is derived, indeed, you can use it as it is. The equation looks like :

$$r_s = 1 - \frac{6 \sum d^2}{N(N^2 - 1)}$$

Research appreciation

Where

> r = Spearmans rank order correlation
> 1 = a constant) These never change
> 6 = a constant   whatever your example
> Σ = the sum of
> d = differences in rank (position in list)
> N = number in group

The easiest way to use the formula is to draw up a table so that you can carry out each step of the equation in turn. In our equation we need to find out:

> d = diff in rank
> d^2 = diff in rank squared

So our table looks like:

Table 7.6

Patient	No of visits	rank/ position	satisfaction score	rank/ position	difference in rank (d)	difference squared (d^2)
1	2	1	3	4	3	9
2	3	2	3	4	2	4
3	5	3	5	1	2	4
4	6	4	4	2	2	4
5	8	5	2	6	1	1
6	9	6	3	4	2	4

There are 6 patients so N = 6

If we substitute our example figures for the symbols in the equation, it looks like:

$$= \frac{1 - 6 \times (9+4+4+4+1+4)}{6(6^2 - 1)}$$
$$= 1 - \frac{6 \times 26}{6(36 - 1)} = 1 - \frac{156}{6 \times 35} = 1 - \frac{156}{6 \times 35}$$
$$= 1 - 0.743 = +0.257$$

There is, therefore, only a relatively weak positive correlation between attendance at out-patients and satisfaction.

What can you do with your data?

One final word before leaving correlations; you will notice that earlier the word 'appears' was used to describe the correlation. This is because you should always try to check that the graph you produced shows a real and not a coincidental (or spurious) relationship.

For example, consider the following. The first impression is that symptoms of dizziness, headache etc appeared to increase the higher a climber went up a mountain, so there seems to be a relationship correlation between the two.

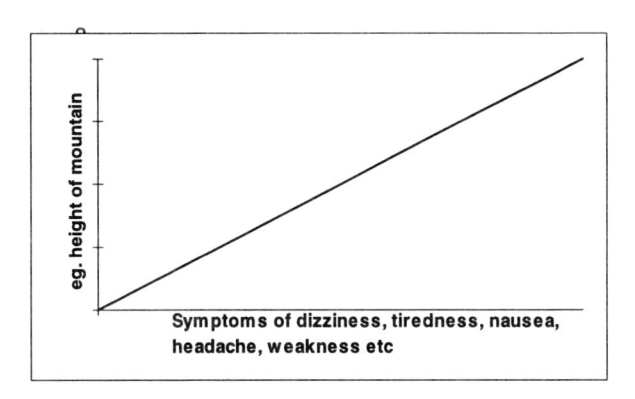

[Graph: y-axis "eg. height of mountain", x-axis "Symptoms of dizziness, tiredness, nausea, headache, weakness etc", showing positive linear relationship]

Figure 7.16

However, we also know that oxygen decreases as we go up a mountain

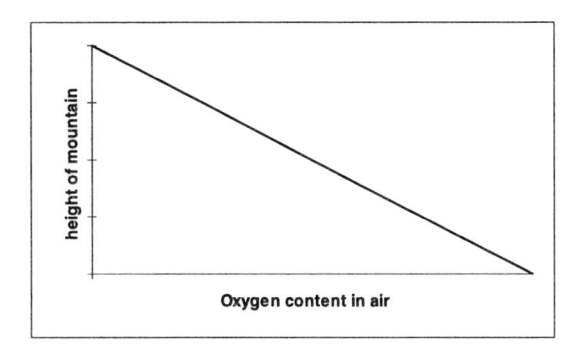

[Graph: y-axis "height of mountain", x-axis "Oxygen content in air", showing negative linear relationship]

Figure 7.17

111

Research appreciation

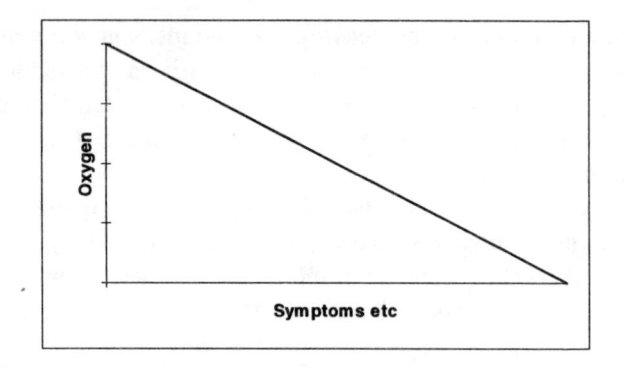

and that lack of oxygten can cause symptoms of dizziness etc.

Figure 7.18

If we give the climber high up on a mountain sufficient oxygen, the symptoms disappear. Thus there is a correlation between oxygen and symptoms and between oxygen and height of the mountain, and there is no real correlation between height of the mountain and symptoms of dizziness. Oxygen is the key variable causing the changes in symptoms.

Always check for key variables by looking for more than one possible correlation/answer from your findings.

Chi square

To complete this chapter on data analysis, we are going to look at one more type of test. As well as the analysis we have discussed, you may wish to see whether differences between groups are real or coincidental and one way to do this, is to use a test of significance. One of the most commonly used tests of significance is chi-square (χ^2).

This test compares the action of groups but can only be used if the particular activity you want to study occurs more than 5 times. It works on the basis that if your groups come from the same or similar samples, then they will have similar trends and tendencies, so what is expected to occur in one group should occur in the other.

What can you do with your data?

You then compare what you expect to happen with what actually did happen.

For example, suppose you were working with two GP group practices and were asked to look at health promotion programmes. Both GPs are concerned about the number of patients who attend well men classes and want to know if one practice has more success with its programme than the other.

In the first practice 100 men attend 200 classes

In the second practice 70 men attend 120 classes

The same programme is offered in both practices but you are unsure whether attendance rates are the same or different as the sample sizes are different.

Again, as with the other tests, chi-square has a set formula/equation which is:

$$\chi^2 = \sum \left[\frac{(O-E)^2}{E} \right]$$

where
- χ^2 = chi square
- Σ = the sum of
- O = what was observed to happen (actual frequency)
- E = what you expected to happen (expected frequency)

So, if we are to act as though the groups are from the same population, the total sample and attendance can be found by simple arithmetic.

Total number = patients from practice 1 + patients from practice 2
= 100 + 70 = 170

Total attendances = attendances at practice 1 + attendances at practice 2
= 200 + 120 = 320

Therefore, if each individual in the total sample behaved in the same way, each would have attended

Research appreciation

The next step is to use this **individual** rate and see how many classes would have been attended in each practice if the groups were behaving in the same way.

Total practice attendance = number of attendances per person
x
number in practice attending

practice 1 = 1.88 x 100 = 188
practice 2 = 1.88 x 70 = 131

We call this result the expected frequency.

Then the easiest way to complete the test is to do as we did with the Spearman rank order correlation and draw up a table showing the working of each stage. This looks like:

Table 7.7

	Expected frequency E	Actual or observed frequency O	O – E	$(O-E)^2$	$\frac{(O-E)^2}{E}$
Practice 1	188	200	12	144	$\frac{144}{188} = 0.76$
Practice 2	131	120	-11	121	$\frac{121}{131} = 0.92$

$$\text{Now, } \chi^2 = \text{the sum of } \frac{(O-E)^2}{E} = 0.76 + 0.92$$
$$= 1.68$$

Chi-squared values are looked up on a special table (see Appendix). If you look at that table you will see that it uses significance levels which we discussed previously, but also degrees of freedom, and before using the table you need to understand what this term means. At school, do you remember being given examples such as:

a + b + c + d = 12

What can you do with your data?

and you had to work out what a, b, c and d were. In fact, a, b and c could be almost any number but d had to be a number that would give the required answer of 12. So, of the four numbers, only **3** can vary freely and we say that in that equation these are 3 degrees of freedom.

In our example there are only two groups, so working on the basis described above, there is **one** degree of freedom.

Look up the answer at one degree of freedom (see x^2 chart on page 114) and we can see that our figure is smaller than those on the table – regardless of significance level. Therefore, we cannot say there is a significant difference between the two groups.

Just one more point, you may wish to compare more than two groups. Suppose there were four practices and not two.

in the first practice 100 men attend 200 classes

in the second practice 70 men attend 120 classes

in the third practice 40 men attend 90 classes

in the fourth practice 85 men attend 150 classes

You would work out the total population as shown before, and then set up a table like table 7.7.

Table 7.8: Attendances at classes

	Expected figures	Actual or observed frequency	O–E	$(O-E)^2$	$\dfrac{(O-E)^2}{E}$
practice 1					
practice 2					
practice 3					
practice 4					

For x^2 with a table like this, we call figures going across rows (e.g. all of practice 1 information = 1 row) and the figures going down columns (e.g. all figures under heading 'Expected figures' make 1 column). Therefore, in our table, we have four rows and two

Research appreciation

columns. Chi square has another standard equation for degrees of freedom where there are more than two variables being compared:

$$df = (rows-1)(columns-1)$$

if you substitute our figure

$$df = (4-1)(2-1)$$
$$= 3$$

Now you try working out this second example. Carry out your sum as shown and look up the answer this time at 3 degrees of freedom (*answer given at the end of the chapter*).

Conclusion

This chapter has only given you an introduction to analysing and presenting data, and you may find you need more information to complete your analysis so some useful texts have been included at the end of the chapter. However, by following all the worked examples and using your figures rather than those given in the chapter, you should be able to present your findings in a clear and easily understood format.

Answer to examples

Answer to Figure 7.4

$$\text{mean deviation} = \frac{10}{5} = 2$$

$$\text{standard deviation} = \sqrt{\frac{47}{5}} = \sqrt{8.4} = 2.89$$

Answer to Figure 7.7

Answer = 5.11 which is smaller than the figure on the x^2 table for 3 df, so again there is no significant difference between the attendances of the group

Additional Reading

Gore S m and Altman D G (1982). *Statistics in Practice*, B M J, London.

Hicks C M (1990). *Research and Statistics. A Practical Introduction for Nurses*, Prentice Hall, Hemel Hempstead.

Huff D (1973). *How to Lie with Statistics*, Penguin, Harmondsworth

Moser C A and Kalton G (1971). *Survey Methods in Social Investigation*, Heinemann, New York.

Oppenheim A N (1990). *Questionnaire Design and Attitude Measurement*, Heinemann, New York.

Chapter 8
How do you interpret Interviews and Observation?

So far we've looked at how you can use the information gained from questionnaires. That is quantitative data and you cannot use the same type of analysis with interview and/or observational data. Instead you have to try to interpret an/or explain your finding using actual examples from your data set. In other words instead of adding all your data and then carrying out tests to look for significant differences and patterns, trends and correlations you have to go through your data with a fine toothcomb searching out the meanings. The processes involved in this are time consuming and exacting but carefully used give a very detailed picture of the issue or setting that you have chosen to study. Let's start by looking at interview data.

Analysing Interviews

Step 1

Your first task is to make sure that all the information that you have gathered can be easily used. So if you have used written notes make sure that they are readable, and where you have used shorthand write the actual meaning out before you forget exactly what each abbreviation stood for. You may feel sure that you will remember the meanings but once you start to analyse your data the interviews can merge together in your mind and then you will find it extremely difficult to analyse accurately.

If you have used a tape recorder, do get all your tapes transcribed. You need to be able to study each interview within the context of all the interviews. To be continually swapping tapes is not only time consuming but leads to inaccuracies because only phrases and not the whole interview is recalled. In an ideal world you would be able to ask someone used to transcribing to type out the interviews for you, but with small scale projects you will probably have to do it yourself. It is important that you allow sufficient time for this because, on average, it will take over two hours for each quarter of an hour of interview.

A finished transcript should look something like Figure 8.1 which is a short section from a semi structured interview. A simple system has been used so that it is easy to identify each speaker and to show pauses in speech (....). Words that you cannot hear no matter how you try are written as ???? and xxxx have been substituted where individuals or places could be identified and confidentiality lost.

Figure 8.1 A Section of a Transcribed Interview of a Discussion on Models of Nursing

Respondent Number 11
Interviews listed as number 1
Respondent listed as number 2

2. *yeah well whichever individuals on at that time it would be nice to see a team using a model to plan care or............*

1. **Yes?**

2   *............it would be nice to think that we could ???? a nursing model and use it for a collaborative care plan. Things like that are going to hopefully going to change anyway*

1. **so what sort of model would you like?**

2   *me, myself? .....erm I suppose something like Roper's with a checklist 'cos that's the good way of teaching with some elements of sort of Orem, that type of model 'cos on xxxxx ward we are meant to be ...uhm an acute area but then a rehabilitation area and that's a suitable model to combine the two...........*

1. **do you see your model being used on other wards?**

2. *well we hadn't really thought that far.... it's a nice idea...I suppose we could...yeah...it would be nice to think so but I*

How do you interpret interviews and observations

mean really it's more really that I...I mean my main objective is to improve our care and therefore the care of the patient as well so it's not an area that needs complication I've spoken to half a dozen or so of the students as well as the rest of the staff and I think we can work out what we actually want... we can want... we can convert a system... it might be basic but it'll be clear.

Step 2

Your next step is to attach any post interview notes (Lofland and Lofland 1984) that you made to the relevant interview notes. Once you are sure that you have gathered all your data you should take two copies of everything and immediately put the original away, unmarked and intact until the end of the project. This is your safety net and is there to provide a full data set should you need the raw data again, or should the data set that you are working on become lost or damaged.

Step 3

Now you can begin the analysis, but you need to consider two things:

1. what you are looking for, and
2. how you find it.

Let us consider point one – what exactly do you look for in interview data? Well, you are going to try to use your data to explain why the people in your study act as they do. A very clear example of this type of analysis is Cornell's (1984) *'Hard Earned Lives'*. This is an exploration of working class womens' attitudes and beliefs about health and is well worth reading if you plan to use interviewing. However, do remember that this was a big, long-term project and you will be working on a much smaller scale.

So, how do you find it? You need to start by sitting and reading through all your transcripts. This is not as easy as it sounds because inevitably the things that you are reading will spark off ideas of patterns and trends. In this initial read through you should jot these down on a separate piece of paper and then, when you have read right through the transcript, you should write a short summary (this helps you to put each interview in context) and attach this to the transcript. When you have gone through all the transcripts it is worth spending ten minutes looking at your jottings and drawing up a full list of the potential patterns and trends. You may need to look at the summaries to help you.

Step 4

Next you need to start a separate file for each of the emerging themes, and this is where the reason for having two working copies of the data (remember you originally took two copies) becomes apparent. While one copy remains intact so that you can always look at the whole interview, the other can be cut up so that all the respondents comments on each theme can be placed in one folder. It is vital at this point to mark on each passage the respondent's number, the page number and the paragraph number (see figure 8.2).

Figure 8.2: An Example of an Extract from an Interview looking at views on record keeping

2. *I'd like to start....I'd like to start them being serious with the documents, I'd like the staff to sign them because I think that they don't need to put down and then they forget the things that are important. I think the fact that they're legal documents makes people aware so they just....tick...you know we have to write down the problems and the background and it's being done without background that's the problem...I mean, like specific nursing care I'd like to see things written down...how they're mobilising, how it's going, how they feel. I think it's important I think our initials should be clear.*
    respondent No 1 page 4, paragraph 2.

This system of cross referencing means that, not only can you study each theme and trend separately and in great detail, you can easily

How do you interpret interviews and observations

altering the meaning of the extract by using it out of context. This is vital because you could bias or totally invalidate your findings by using passages injudiciously. Also, if you do not have such a thorough system, you can waste hours of time trying to find who said what, and where it was in the transcript.

Step 5 So, back to your first folder and read all the extracts again, create a mind map by brainstorming all the issues raised within this one theme. For example, if your theme was anger and within that five issues were raised, you could draw a flow chart as in figure 8.3.

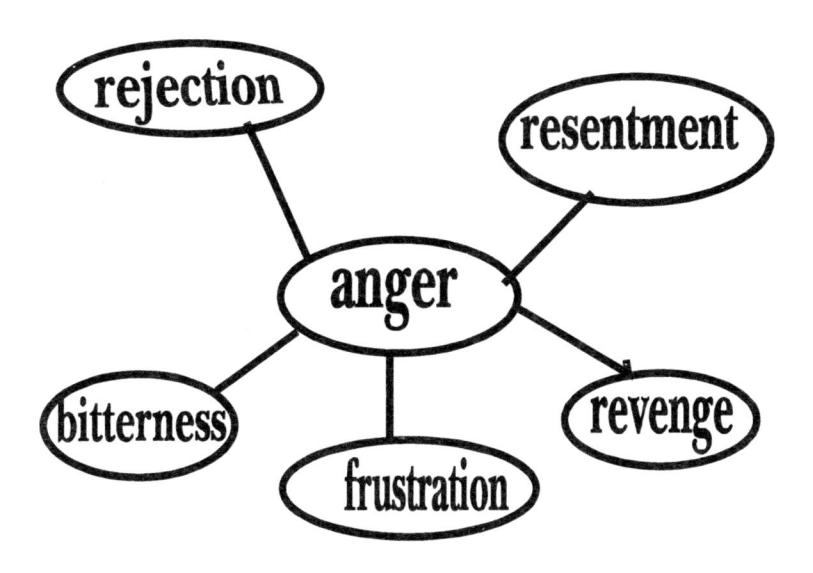

Figure 8.3 Flow chart showing Mind Map

Your next step would be to look at the extracts and see how often these issues arose in each interview. You do this by creating a grid as follows.

123

Table 8.1: Grid

Theme anger	interview 1	interview 2	interview 3	interview 4
at rejection	p1, p7, p11	p4	p2, p6, p6	p1, p4, p10
at authority	p2, p8, p9	p1, p3, p5, p6	p4, p7, p8	p1, p3, p8

This type of grid gives you an idea of how often each issue arose in each individual interview and in the project as a whole, and the importance you will give to each issue in your discussion. Once you have done this you then start to link the issues together and write your own description and discussion of your findings showing how the issues support and explain the main theme identified.

You follow this process for each folder/theme in turn.

Step 6

As you will realise by now there is no quick way to analyse interview data, it takes time and patience, because the final step is to check and recheck your findings.

Once you are confident that you have identified a theme, pattern or specific issue you need to check that you have not added in your own attitudes and values as this will affect the accuracy of your results. For example, you may think that the respondent meant more than they actually said (English is a language where understatement is often used), or that they were exaggerating. You cannot comment on this you can only use the information you have gathered and whilst you may comment that one particular interview differs from all the others you cannot give the respondents rationale for what they said.

Similarly you may think that respondents who gave similar answers were definitely agreeing with each other. This is not the case. Each one was talking to you, so you can discuss the similarity and consistency of your findings but you cannot infer anything more. Ascribing meanings that you cannot substantiate will invalidate your study. You must make sure that your readers know that, whilst there seemed to be consensus in some areas, further study would be needed to ascertain whether these were real or coincidental similarities.

Part of final stage is to check that you have recognised the way in which the target population used language, as meanings and interpretations of words vary considerably (Phillips 1981). If your interviews include respondents from different classes, parts of the country or cultural backgrounds, particularly where English is not the first language you need to take this into account in your use of the data. Failure to do so would bias your results.

Step 7

To summarise the function of interview data is to illuminate and interpret. It is not usually quantifiable but instead provides a wealth of data than can be used to identify an indication of a particular event, practice, attitude or belief. It can be used as the pilot for a much bigger study (or survey) which is quantifiable, or as the follow on to a survey to try to explain the findings.

Observational data

This third type of data is different again, here if you think back to chapter six you are trying to describe a social setting, or understand how and why a particular group acts as it does. A good example of this kind of work is Brown's (1989) 'Individualised care: The Role of the Ward Sister', but again you need to remember that her project was much bigger than the projects that you are likely to undertake. However it has very useful pointers for you when analysing your own data.

The different types of observation provide different data sets, so each will be considered separately.

Nonparticipant Observation

The whole idea of this kind of project is to provide a detailed or even exhaustive description of a particular setting. You will have gathered piles of information which may at first appear incomprehensible see table 8.2.

Research appreciation

Table 8.2: Analysis of observations inInteractions at chosen (key) places

Place	Time in seconds				
	0-5	6-10	11-15	16-20	21-25
Reception desk	^{1}A1 ^{1}A5	^{4}B5	^{2}B5	^{1}A6	^{2}A1
Weighing scales	^{2}A2	^{3}A1 ^{3}A2	^{5}A2	^{4}A3 ^{4}A2	^{5}A2
Waiting chairs (give chair and patient a number)	^{4}B2 ^{3}B2	^{2}B3	^{1}B2 ^{1}A3	^{1}A3 ^{1}B3	^{4}A3
Door from consulting room	^{3}A4	^{5}B1 ^{1}A1	^{2}A3	^{3}B4 ^{3}A4	^{1}A4
Door out of clinic	^{5}A2	^{1}A3	\	^{2}B1	\

However, remember that it was you who designed the categories that you have used (as discussed in Chapter 6) so given time and patience you will be able to work through your findings and begin to describe the setting. The additional notes taken at the end of the session will help in this process and Spradley (1980) suggests there are three categories that can be used to help categorise data for analysis, these are:

1: Descriptive observation: This category is designed with basic aim of providing a clear description of the place, people and events that took place. For instance using the example cited in chapter six of an outpatient clinic, this data would include the description of the layout of the clinic, the numbers of staff, whether they wore uniform, the number of patients, where they sat etc. This can be used to provide the basis for future observations.

2. Focused Observations: These are often based on descriptive observations which have been used to provide an overview of the whole setting and enable the researcher to see which area he/she wishes to concentrate or focus on. Using your first descriptive results you decide exactly which of your observation you wish to concentrate on. In other words which aspects of the situation will allow you to explore the main issues of the project.

3. Selective Observations: These are really just observations that are even more specific than the focused data and these you will usually have collected towards the end of your period of field work because the longer you observe the more familiar you become with the phenomena you are studying and the more sure you are of the type of information that you need.

Once you have decided which pattern and trends are emerging from your data you can look back at the interactions that you found before the project started and see how this links with your findings.

It may be that previous research supports your findings, or alternatively you may have found something different. Remember observation is like a photograph and you see what happened at any given point in time but there is **no** explanation as to why it happened and you **must not** try to state why things happened. You do not know. This method of data collection and analysis is only designed to help you analyse **what** happened. If you want to know **why** it happened you must use another method as well (e.g. interviews).

However, sometimes all you need is the picture. In our example we chose to look at an outpatient clinic; the picture provided shows what is happening. If the interactions/activities found in this example are not satisfactory then you need to think about ways to improve things. So the observation is vital, it provides the starting point, it enables you to *'see the clinic'* again and devise ways to improve the service offered. This can then be discussed with those involved and, if appropriate, implemented.

Participant observation

The aim of this type of project is to provide an in depth analysis of the actions and activities of a particular group. In Chapter 6, we discussed the way to collect data using field notes and then transcribing these and adding notes about the session as a whole.

You will find you have an immense amount of data and the easiest way to analyse this is to follow similar guidelines to those given earlier in this chapter for analysing interview data.

You should start by reading through notes for each block of time and then noting the recurrent activities and actions that occur. The next step is to construct a grid, clearly identifying who, when and how these activities and actions occur. This type of systematic analysis is important because memory is selective and you may think an activity occurs often when, in fact, it occurs infrequently but the surrounding activities are such that the activity appears prominent. Similarly, other actions that appear as minor may be found to occur with surprising frequency.

Brainstorming and mind maps may help as you try to discuss and describe your findings. Remember to try to use discussion with group members to explain and interpret actions, and not just your own perceptions. It is easy to use your views to override those of group members because you will have become immersed in the group. However, although you know the group extremely well and may identify with them, your mores and values will be different to theirs and can influence your analysis, preventing you from giving an accurate interpretation.

If you accept and recognise your biases, you can use participant observation to present a view and understanding of a particular group that could not be found in any other way. However, in nursing and health care, full participant observation may not be appropriate or possible and you may prefer to use this approach to data collection but act as participant as observer. The difference here is that, initially, the group are aware that you, although a participant, will be studying specific activities or actions. As with participant observation, this is not a short-term study because you need to wait until the group have accepted you (or perhaps your changed role) and have relaxed again. However, for many health care professions, the fact that the group is aware of the proposed study initially makes the approach more ethically acceptable.

References

Brown R (1989). *Individual care: The Role of The Ward Sister*, RCN, Scutari Press, London

Burgess RG (ed) (1982). *Field Research A Sourcebook and Field Manual*, Unwin Hyman, London.

Burgess R G (1984). *In the Field*, Unwin Hyman, London.

Cornell J (1984). *Hard Earned Lives*,

Lofland F, Lofland J (1984) *Analysing Social Settings*,

Phillips D R (1981). *Do-It-Yourself Social Surveys*, The Polytechnic of North London.

Spradley J P (1980). *Participant Observation*, Holt Rhinehart and Winston, New York.

Chapter 9
How Do You Write about It?

The report of a project is an important as the project itself! If no reports were written then we would spend all our time going over ground already covered.

The purpose of any report is to disseminate knowledge in a format that can be understood and utilised by others, - whether the findings are as you expected, whether the project had major problems concerned with design or analysis or whether the project substantiates the findings of other workers it can be used by peers and students.

Research reports therefore need to consider certain elements.

The Audience

Before you start to write you need to consider first and foremost for whom the report is intended. Professionals, academics, clients/patients or the general public. All will have different requirements and you may find that you need to consider writing more than one type of report.

Generally speaking academic and/or professional reports are the most demanding and those for the general public the most straight forward. However it is essential that you remember if writing for client or the public you must not write in such a way that individuals' expectations are raised in a way that cannot be met.

Whichever audience you are writing for do not use jargon. Any specific terms that you use should be explained either in the text or in an accompanying glossary of terms. The most common mistake in research reports is the belief that the reader understands the terms used. This may be true but it is more usual to find that the reader has an imperfect understanding and therefore the whole report can be misunderstood purely because the true context is not clear.

You want your chosen audience to read what you have written and not either fall asleep from boredom or give up because they are hopelessly confused or lost in the welter of data presented. You must therefore organise your report carefully both in content and layout, so that the reader finds a clear logical account of what actually happened (not what you hoped would happen). Research is planned, systematic and follows procedural guidelines so it should be possible to visualise the stages of the project just from reading about it.

The Title

In todays increasingly technological world where literature searches are conducted with systems that only use titles you must choose words that give some clue to the project content. Catchy titles may appeal and may have their uses in publishing but if they give no indication of the subject matter that project may well be overlooked.

The title can be generalistic e.g. A study of nu*rses undergoing post-registration training courses* or specific, e.g. *A study of four women with bulimia*.

If you are determined to have a catchy title then it should be short and should be followed by a definitive description as in the two examples above. That way potential readers can decide whether the project is pertinent to their own studies.

The Abstract

This is a short summary of the project usually between 100-200 words in length. It goes at the front of the project and allows the reader to make an informed choice as to whether to read the whole project. It is worth noting that in some cases abstracts are published in collections to help other researchers in the same field for example, nursing abstracts and sociological abstracts.

The abstract should be organised so that the first sentence gives a clear statement of the problem/situation that you investigated. This should be followed by a brief outline of the research methodology and sampling technique used. It concludes with a short summary of the findings and conclusions.

For example:

> *This study was carried out on an acute surgical ward, the aim was to establish whether different regimes for mobilisation following major surgery affected the recovery of patients. The research focused on the two programmes, how these were implemented and how the patients saw their care. Data was collected using two methods, nonparticipant observation conducted over a three week period, and semi-structured interviews. Patients were observed following surgery using diary records and time sampling. Interviews were conducted with both patients and staff and the interview data compared with the observational findings. Analysis of the observational data showed one programme appeared to be more effective. The interview data also showed a clear preference of staff for that method, and patients experiencing that programme also expressed a higher level of satisfaction with their care. Whilst this was only a small study, the consistency of the findings suggests that there are implications for patient care that arise from this study.*

Introduction

This should be a general discussion of the background to the project and its potential importance and benefits. You may wish to state why you should undertake the project ie. why you background made you particularly suited to this project.

You should give some indication of definitive work in your field or if this is an unresearched field you should discuss why it has been under-researched and how the lack of available data has affected the study design. You should also briefly discuss any policy implications that may arise as a result of your study. Finally, you should also include a general discussion of the hypothesis, statement or question.

In other words the purpose of this section is to set the scene for the whole project.

Background Literature

This section is perfectly straight forward and is, as it suggests, a discussion (or review) of relevant research in the field. This is the theoretical background to the study, it is said to 'inform the project', where different aspects of the subject are to be studied you may wish to subdivide the total review into 5 or 6 sections. If you do this you should state that you are going to do so in a short introduction at the start of this section.

Methodology

This is a very important chapter in any report as it is on this section that validity of the study will be judged, as will the ability to apply the findings (the generalisability) to the population. It should provide sufficient detail for another researcher to design and set up a similar project. It should be sub-divided so that the reader can clearly see.

i) the hypothesis, statement or question that is to be studied.

ii) the method chosen including the strength, weaknesses or limitations of the method chosen. You should back up your choice with recognised texts.

iii) the type and size of the sample and how potential respondents were contacted.

iv) the design of the tool (questionnaire, schedule, field, notes etc) together with an indication of the measurement devices used e.g. Likert scales.

v) how the project was operationalised. This should include discussion of any pilot study and the resulting modification of the project tool.

vi) how the resulting data was analysed.

vii) the ethical issues involved, including specific areas such as confidentiality as well as the more theoretical concepts involved in health service research.

Results

This chapter in the report should be a clear presentation of the actual data gathered. It is only intended to show the unedited findings and should not be used as a discussion of these.

Remember that although you may find it fascinating there is nothing more off-putting than pages and pages of figures. Try to think of ways to make the data immediately clear to the reader. Use pie charts, bar charts, histograms and graphs as well as tables. Do not try to cram too much data into any one table or chart and always explain each illustration. If you include data and do not explain it properly readers cannot accurately assess your findings.

Choose the key findings of the study and make sure that these stand out and cannot be overlooked.

State clearly if you have collected more than one kind of data and present each type under separate sub-sections. Note that in some interpretive studies this section is limited as discussion of specific points may be an essential part of the presentation. Where this is the case then you must ensure that a logical profession through the data is still possible.

Discussion

As the title of this chapter suggest this is the section in which you can discuss in detail the findings of your study, referring back to the literature. The hypothesis, statement or question which you have tested should be clearly related to relevant data and fully discussed.

The broader implications of the study should also be discussed and these could include policy, practice and/or training.

The limitations of the study together with any major problems that arose and may affected the validity of the project should be honestly stated and briefly discussed.

It is not unusual for projects to raise new questions. If this happens these should be mentioned and an indication of how they arose during the project should be given, together with a theoretically backed argument as to why they are questions that need addressing.

Conclusion

This should be a summary of the major findings, uses and limitations of the project as a whole. Any new issues should be mentioned and where possible suggestions for future projects should be made. Any major gaps in the findings should be commented on as should any methodological difficulties that may have affected the findings.

Referencing

This should be standard throughout the project. Always check which system is to be used. Harvard is easier when you are not used to writing reports, but it really doesn't matter provided you do not change systems part way through.

Appendices

Always keep a copy of any schedules, questionnaires, field-notes etc used as you may wish to include these as an appendix to your report. This is essential when writing for professional and/or academic audiences.

Useful Reading

Bell (1987). *Doing Your Own Research Project*, Open University Press, Milton Keynes

Chapter 10
Glossary of Research Terms

This glossary has been set alphabetically, but in statistics terms are often put together and you may need to refer to other parts of the glossary in order to fully understand some of the definitions.

Alternative
Hypothesis............This is also called experimental hypothesis, sometimes researchers use this in statistical tests to try to reject the null hypothesis

Bias......................1. In a questionnaire/schedule it is caused by inappropriate or leading questions
2. In a sample it means that the sample being used is not representative of the total population so generalisations should not be made

Case......................An individual within the sample being studied

Causal Link...........A causal link is generally accepted as occurring if one event or factor (A) is shown to have an effect on another (B)

Central
Tendency..............The central tendency is the overall term used to describe the different ways to measure the 'average' of a set of figures ie, the mean, median and the mode

Chi-Square............The comparison of the number of times that something actually occurs (the actual frequency) with the number of times that it's expected to occur (the expected frequency) note chi-square should not be used with very small numbers and where something is expected to occur less than 5 times.

Research appreciation

Closed
Question ....A question where respondents can only answer using previously decided categories eg. yes, no.

Coding....................A method of analysis where all answers to questions are put into specific categories and then studied for inter-relationships. Large scale surveys often used pre-coded questionnaires

Coefficient of
Correlation ....The amount of relationship between any two sets of scores or cases. It is based on the assumption that the relationship between the variables is adequately described by a straight line, numerically it lies between +1.0 (a perfect relationship) and -1.0 (a perfect negative relationship)

Confidence
Interval ....Indicates the range within the normal curve of distribution within which a particular value lies. It is calculated by working in both directions from the mean of a normal curve of distribution, and is usually written as a definite number ± another much smaller number eg.24 ± 3

Correlation ....The relationship between two variables. Note - it is possible to get a correlation without there being a direct causal link between variables either by chance or because both have a relationship with a third variable.

Correlation
Study ....A study only concerned with investigating the relationship/ association between variables

Critical Case...........Where an individual or group are seen as especially significant for a particular study.

Cross
Tabulation. ....A statistical measure whereby two variables are graphically plotted against one another.

Glossary of research terms

Curves of
Distribution ....The graphical presentation of data showing where most observations are grouped, there are several different types of curve.

    1. Normal Curve of Distribution. Sometimes called the Gaussian curve is the systematic distribution of observations round a central point. Most samples drawn from the population as a whole tend to follow the same pattern, hence the term, 'normal'

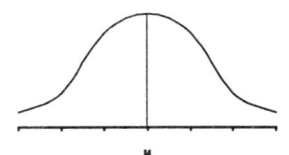

Degrees of
Freedom ....Numerically equal to the number of changes that can be made to a group of scores or cases whilst satisfying external constraints eg. if 4 + 3 +2 + 3 = 12 -only three of the numbers can change - the fourth has to ensure the final number is 12, so in this case there are 3 degrees of freedom - sometimes written as (N-1) where N = total number of scores or cases.

Empirical
Research. ....The systematic collection of data

Field-notes.............Detailed notes taken of a social setting by a researcher undertaking qualitative research

Forced
choice scale ....A scale used in questionnaires where respondents are given a range of choices, but where there is no don't know/unsure category. ie.respondents are forced to make a choice either positively or negatively.

Frequency
Distribution .... Shows the frequency with which each value in the sample occurs (usually shown in tabular or diagrammatic form)

Grounded
Theory .... A theory that offers an explanation of social phenomena based on data that has been gathered and analysed using a process of induction, deduction and verification.

Histogram .... Also called a bar chart, a method of presenting data where each category of data is presented as a block.

Hypothesis .... A proposition put forward by a researcher which is evaluated using empirical data.

Independent
Variable .... The variable or conditions that the researcher alters or manipulates during a project.

Interval Data .... A type of measurement scale where the individual values are distinguishable, ordered and where the intervals between each point on the scale are equal.

Likert Scale .... A scale used in questionnaires where respondents are given a range of possible answers eg. strongly agree, agree, disagree, strongly disagree, not sure/don't know.

Mean .... Probably the most commonly used measure of central tendency, - like the balance point on a see-saw it is the point of balance of a set of scores. Found by adding up the values of all the scores and dividing by the number of scores in the set. eg. 5+6+3+4 mean = 4.5

Median .... A measure of central tendency found by listing the scores in order of rank, the median is the middle score.

Methodology .... This term has two meanings:

Glossary of research terms

        1. The methods by which data can be collected eg. interview

        2. the study of the methods used in projects

Mode .... The third measure of central tendency but in this case the measure is the most frequently occurring value. eg. if ten people take a test and four have the same mark while all the others differ the mark occurring four times is the mode.

Nominal data .... The simplest scale and used when all that can be said about the data is that all categories are mutually exclusive and individual scores or cases can only fit into one category eg. particular religious sects.

Null hypothesis ..... Is used when comparing two sample means. The assumption that is made is that the two samples are from the same (or identical) populations. Therefore there is no statistical difference between the samples.

Non-participant Observation. .... A method whereby the researcher observes a social setting but takes no part at all in the actions/inter-actions of the group being studied.

Participant Observation .... A research strategy where the researcher is actively involved in the social setting that is being researched. Where the researcher is fully involved in the setting in order to experience its characteristics the strategy is referred to as complete participation

Probability .... The change of likelihood of something occurring, based on repeated observations.

Ratio Scale .... The values are ranked, the points on the scale or equidistant and there is an absolute or non-arbitrary zero, eg. metres and kilograms.

Research appreciation

Reliability..............The extent to which a test, measurement or means of data collection can be reproduced in other studies.

Sampling
Distribution...........Curve of distribution formed by plotting the means of different samples.

Scattergram............A graph showing the relationship between variables, where each point represents a separate case.

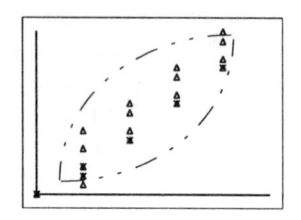

Significance
Level......................This is the probability of making a type I error (rejecting assumptions that are in fact true) and it can be set at any desired level (eg.5%) provided the sampling is continuous.

Standard
Deviation...............A measurement which shows how much the scores or cases taken together (as a whole group) deviate from the mean.

Triangulation..........The term when a researcher uses more than one methodology in a particular project.

Validity..................The extent to which a test measures what it is supposed to measure.

Variable.................A characteristic, attribute or property that varies, eg. gender, age, sex.

Variance................The square of the standard deviation used by statisticians as it avoids the problems caused by negative deviations from the mean cancelling out the corresponding positive ones.

Appendix I

Referencing your work

The idea of referencing your work is to enable readers to:
1. Identify all the sources of material that you have used.
2. Assess whether you have made appropriate use of source material to present a reasoned logical argument. That means you have not just linked the various pieces of information together. You have. in fact, used your sources to illustrate and explain the subject under discussion.
3. Recognise and understand the focus of your work.
4. Consider the material that you have presented as acceptable evidence that supports/disproves a particular point of view.
5. Check the origin and accuracy of your sources.
6. Locate and follow up material of interest.

There are several different systems of referencing. This book uses the Harvard system and although initially, it may appear confusing, using a standard system for referencing is easy once you are used to it. Listed below are some simple guidelines to help you with this system.

There are two places where references should be used:
- a) in the text
- b) at the end of your piece of work

If you wish to use an author whose whole research presents a particular argument or viewpoint, you should use phrases such as:

Smith (1989) argues that....or
Smith (1989) suggests...........

If the information that you are presenting is not just the overall theme but can be pin-pointed to a certain part of the work, you should extend the referencing and identify the page where the actual argument/statement is made, so:

Smith (1989:24) argues that..........or
Smith (1989:24) points out.........

If you are including a direct quote to reinforce your discussion, the length of the quote will affect how your write it.

a) a short quote of three to four words should be written in the text but marked with quotation marks as well as the details given when the overall argument/findings are used

Smith (1989:24) writes '................' or

According to Smith (1989:24) '..............' or

'......................' Smith (1989:24)

b) a long quote should be set out separately in a clear indented paragraph followed by the usual details:

....
....
....
....
....
....' *(Smith 1989:24)*

If your quote finishes towards the end of the indented line, write the details underneath:

'..
....
....
....
....

Smith (1989:24)

Whenever you indent a paragraph, always leave at least one line above and below the quote so that it stands out clearly and does not appear to be part of the overall text.

Remember the year that you quote is the year that the edition you have used was published. The number of the edition (if any) is given at the front of the book. If the word 'impression' is used followed by a date, this does not mean the same as edition and should not be used instead of the year of edition.

When an author has published more than one book in any one year, it is customary to put a small letter after the year, so:

Smith (1989a:24)

Smith (1989b:24)

Appendix I

When an author has contributed a chapter to a book edited by someone else, it is usual to refer to the author in the text either by:
>as Smith discusses..............................in Brown (1990:26) or
>in Smith's view.................................(Brown 1990:26)

Where a publication has been written by two authors, both should be quoted in the text:
>Smith and Jones (1989:45)

Where more than two authors are involved, you do not need to write all the names out in the text. Instead you can put:
>Smith *et al* (1989:45)

At the end of each piece of work, the following information should be given:
>Surname of Author
>Initials of Author
>Year of Publication
>Title of Publication
>Publisher
>Place of Publication

Authors' surnames should be recorded alphabetically.

Where the *'et al'* convention has been used, it is customary to list all the authors full details:

Book publications should be set out as follows:
>Smith J (1989). <u>Understanding Poverty</u>, Pelican, London

Journal publications should be set out as follows:
>Smith J (1989). Understanding Poverty, "<u>Community Care</u>", Vol. 10, Number 7, p 271-76

Notice the difference in underlining and the inclusion of quotation marks for the journal publication, as well as the additional information about the journal.

Editors should be acknowledged by the letters (Ed) after the name:
>Smith J (Ed) (1989). <u>Understanding Poverty</u>, Pelican, London
>Jones A (1989). "Unemployment", in <u>Understanding Poverty</u>, Smith J (Ed), Pelican, London

Finally, the list of references should include all materials referred to in the text, whilst the bibliography includes all the background reading not necessarily quoted.

Tips:

Try to collect useful words and phrases such as 'suggests that'; 'argues'; 'points out'; 'describes'; 'goes on to' etc.

Try to avoid using 'I' and instead use objective phrases such as 'it has been suggested'; 'practical experience may show' etc.

Table for Chi Square

Degrees of Freedom	0.05	0.01	Degrees of Freedom	0.05	0.01
1	3.84	6.63	16	26.30	32.00
2	5.99	9.21	17	27.59	33.41
3	7.81	11.34	18	28.87	34.81
4	9.49	13.28	19	30.14	36.19
5	11.07	15.09	20	31.41	37.57
6	12.59	16.81	21	32.67	38.93
7	14.07	18.48	22	33.92	40.29
8	15.50	20.09	23	35.17	41.64
9	16.90	21.67	24	36.42	42.98
10	18.31	23.21	25	37.65	44.31
11	19.68	24.72	26	38.89	45.64
12	21.03	26.22	27	40.11	46.96
13	22.36	27.69	28	41.34	48.28
14	23.68	29.14	29	42.56	49.59
15	25.00	30.58	30	43.77	50.89

Useful Symbols and Abbreviations

A .... acual results
d .... 1. deviation of a score or case from the mean
            2. difference between two scores
df .... degrees of freedom
E .... expected results
f .... frequency of scores within an interval
M .... the mean
N .... the number of individuals, scores or cases in the sample
p .... probability
q .... quantity
r .... correlation coefficient
r_s .... Spearman rank order correlation
S .... sample
S_M .... sample mean
SD .... standard deviation of a sample
> .... greater than
< .... less than
x_1 .... an individual score or case
x .... a particular score or case
$\bar{x}$ .... mean
y .... any score or case other than x
χ^2 .... chi-square (test for significant differences)
φ .... phi
σ .... sigma (variance)
Σ .... the sum of

Index

costs of research 23–25
courses - diploma/degree 27
data - types of 6, 94
- analysis of 94
- numerical analysis- levels of measurement 81–117
- ordinal scales 82
- interval scales 82
- ratio scales 83
-averages 83–4
- standard deviation 94–117
- analysis of interview data 115–125
-analysis of observation data 119-22
- presentation of 85–117
   pie charts 88
   bar charts 90, 91
   graphs 92, 93
data collection 43–79
- interviewing 68–71
- observation 72–79
- surveys 61–68
- triangulation 6
- questionnaire design 61–68

ethics in research 7,62-5,92

funding research 27-31

glossary of research terms 135–142

hypothesis 5

interviewing 68–71
- stuctured interviewing 69
- semistructured 69
- unstructured 70

libraries, types of 27
   sources of
- information in 26–32
literature reviewing 6, 35–41
literature searching 35–41

observation 72–79
- non-participation 72–78
- participant 78–79

research protocol, developing 9-14
research question, developing 17–23

sample 7
sampling 43–53
- sampling frames 43–46
- sample size 46
- types of sample 46–53

writing a literature review 35–42
writing a report 126–131

149